Osteopathic Considerations in Systemic Dysfunction

Michael Kuchera, D.O., F.A.A.O.
William Kuchera, D.O., F.A.A.O.

Greyden Press, LLC
Dayton, Ohio

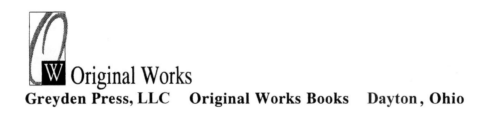 Original Works

Greyden Press, LLC   Original Works Books   Dayton, Ohio

Osteopathic Considerations in Systemic Dysfunction

ISBN 1-57074-154-9

Printer/ Binder: Greyden Press, LLC

"Osteopathic physicians must be able to give a reason for the treatment they give, not so much to the patient, but to themselves."[1]

A.T. Still, M.D.

"The inevitable result of the rapid strides in the study of bacteriology, and pathologic change in tissues and secretions, and the comparatively slow progress which has been made in studying the patient, has been an undue emphasis of the importance of the disease, and a minimizing of the importance of the patient who has it. The dawning of a better day in medicine, however, is now evident . . ."[2]

F.M. Pottenger, M.D.

"(Neuroscience) studies are establishing the physiological bases for determination in man of the visceral consequences of spinal syndromes for which manipulative therapy is advocated."[3]

Horace W. Magoun, Ph.D.

1. Truhlar RE Doctor A.T. Still in the Living. Cleveland, privately printed, 1950, p 112.
2. Pottenger FM Symptoms of Visceral Disease. St Louis, CV Mosby Co, 7th ed, 1953, p 34.
3. Magoun HW: Neuroscience studies in Goldstein M (ed) The Research Status of Spinal Manipulative Therapy, Bethesda MD, US Department of Health, Education and Welfare (NINCDS Monograph #15), 1975, p 210.

FOREWORD

Osteopathy is relatively a young profession in the history of medicine. Slightly over 100 years ago, A.T. Still introduced his philosophy of medical care to the world. The first school of osteopathy was established in Kirksville, Missouri in 1892. It was in this same time period that the germ theory was proposed and eventually the allopathic profession adopted the perspective that this was "the answer to all disease processes." With the discovery of Salversan and eventually penicillin, the allopathic profession launched into an all-out effort to find medicines which would be the "magic bullets." The germ theory of disease promoted the concept that health would be restored and secure if the offending "germ" was found and medically removed.

Because of this majority perspective there are thousands of articles and texts reporting experiences and trials in the use of medications for the treatment of systemic diseases. On the other hand there is relatively little published about augmenting homeostasis or treating host factors in systemic diseases. This text was written to augment the latter category and stresses the structure and function that are pertinent to this perspective. Without specific knowledge of anatomy and physiology, the osteopathic approach would become too "time consuming" and would not be financially feasible to offer a patient with systemic disease.

Osteopathic physicians are educated to use and understand all current medications and surgical procedures for the purpose of promoting health, fighting the disease and supporting the host's physiology. Palpatory and manipulative skills can be used effectively as well as efficiently to aid in diagnosis and treatment of patients with systemic disease or dysfunction.

This text has been divided into several sections in order to present an osteopathic approach to dysfunction manifesting in a particular system or pertinent to a common clinical presentation. These divisions have been primarily grouped by their common autonomic and lymphatic elements but the physician must not be limited to management of the patient within a given system (or section of this text). Because each patient is a unit, dysfunction or disease affecting one part can have far-reaching manifestations.

This text does not propose to replace the many reference texts of medicine and does not include a complete differential diagnosis or a complete treatment plan for the clinical situations that are discussed. Its purpose is to explore selected structural and functional considerations which may produce symptoms or compromise homeostasis. It also demonstrates, by example, clinical application of the osteopathic philosophy in selected situations. Lastly, it attempts to show where osteopathic manipulative treatments can be prescribed as primary or adjunctive modalities available to the D.O. as they assist patients in reaching their maximum health potential.

Even if the patient does not have specific joint somatic dysfunction, manipulative management can be designed to address the following goals:

o .. support the patient's body systems that will be stressed by the
       pathophysiology of the disease
o .. support the patient's natural protective and homeostatic reactions to disease
o .. neutralize detrimental responses of the patient's body to the disease process
o .. provide a synergistic and physiologic approach to the patient's medical
       and/or surgical management
o .. provide a rapid and long-lasting benefit toward improving the patient's level
       of health and immediate comfort

Dysfunction of the soma and its related elements plays a significant role in the production of a variety of patient complaints, signs, and/or symptoms and frequently accompanies underlying visceral dysfunction. For these reasons, palpation for somatic dysfunction is an important part of an osteopathic approach to making a differential diagnosis and it provides essential data for developing a rational total treatment program for the patient. Because osteopathic manipulative treatment is designed to treat the patient's soma and/or to support systemic protective and homeostatic mechanisms, a therapeutic trial of manipulation which addresses the patient's somatic component is an important part of a rational treatment protocol for each patient's visit.

By studying anatomy and physiology from the philosophical vantage point needed to formulate "rational osteopathic treatment," the osteopathic student discovers a unique and valuable perspective of health and disease. Interpretation of somatic clues through understanding of the physiology underlying symptom development allows the physician to surmise the dysfunction or pathophysiology occurring in a given individual patient and offers valuable direction and information for the physical examination and the differential diagnosis. Rather than simply diagnosing and treating symptoms or symptom complexes, the osteopathic physician seeks to augment the health that is found within the individual.

The following relevant comments are found in Pottenger's <u>Symptoms of Visceral Disease</u>[1]:

> "Variability of symptoms is the rule in clinical medicine, a fact which can be readily appreciated by understanding the nerve and chemical control of physiologic function and the factors which influence them, both physical and psychic."

> "It is not only necessary to understand that symptoms produced by a given disease may differ in different individuals and in the same individual at different times, but it is equally necessary to bear in mind that while the stimulus which would be expected to produce a given symptom is present, the symptom may not appear or its reverse may appear if the stimulus to the nerve is excessive, or the neuron itself is hyperexcitable or a certain ionic concentration exists in the body cells. It is necessary, therefore, always to bear in mind that inflammation in organs gives origin to stimuli which have a tendency to produce such and such symptoms, although the symptoms themselves may not materialize."

> "Most of the important symptoms arising from diseases of internal viscera are reflex in nature. In order to understand these symptoms, one must study the innervation of the various viscera and the interrelationship which exists between them, also the interrelationship which exists between the viscera and the skeletal structures."

This text encourages the reader to reexamine familiar medical facts, anatomic relationships and physiologic functions from the osteopathic perspective. This perspective can then be carried into the diagnostic and therapeutic decisions which will repeatedly be required of the medical student and the osteopathic physician for the rest of their professional lives.

---

1. Pottenger FM <u>Symptoms of Visceral Disease</u>. St Louis, CV Mosby Co, 7th ed, 1953, 140.

TABLE OF CONTENTS

INDEX OF FIGURES

INDEX OF TABLES

"My object is to make the Osteopath a philosopher, and place him on the rock of reason."

--A.T. Still, M.D.

OSTEOPATHIC CONSIDERATIONS IN EENT DYSFUNCTION

"All allergic manifestations have a 3-fold etiology: heredity, the allergen, and the structural problem, which is the most fundamental because it lowers resistance and invites malfunction. While nothing can be done about heredity, resistance may be built up to the allergen or it may be avoided. The basic approach is through structure."[1]

I. INTRODUCTION

A wide variety of symptoms and signs referable to the eyes, ears, nose, and/or throat (EENT) will be presented by the patients seen in a busy general practice. EENT pain and/or dysfunction as either a presenting complaint or as a finding of the clinical history and/or physical examination needs careful and thoughtful evaluation by the generalist. The osteopathic practitioner combines somatic palpatory clues and the knowledge of the interrelationships between structure and function with a thorough history and a directed physical examination of the EENT.

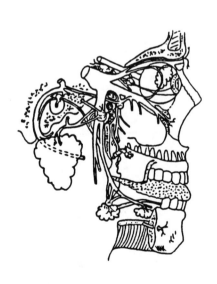

Osteopathic manipulative treatment to the somatic component and considerations toward enhancing body homeostatic mechanisms can play a significant role in designing effective treatment for these patients. Often a successful therapeutic trial with OMT directed at localized dysfunctional states will eliminate the need for systemic treatment or for a more extensive and expensive work-up seeking a non-existent systemic etiology.

Common presenting symptoms or conditions in the EENT system are presented in this section for inclusion in differential diagnosis and treatment design. The somatic component or dysfunctional state occurring with each clinical example is representative of dysfunction in that region.

Because of the interrelationship between structure and function, the presence of dysfunction does not eliminate the possibility of coexisting structural etiologies.

II. PATHOPHYSIOLOGY

REFLEX CONNECTIONS:

Because of a variety of reflex connections, impulses arising from EENT tissues can produce symptoms or dysfunctional states in other structures.[2] Asthma, cephalgia and vertigo are all symptoms which may result from nasal and sinus affections. Stimulation of vagal afferents by the irritation of a plug of wax lodged against the tympanic membrane is clinically associated with a recurrent cough reflex[3] or with dizziness.[4] Both of these symptoms disappear when the wax-irritant is removed.

Impulses originating from outside the EENT may also initiate EENT symptoms because of reflex connections: Cough and hoarseness may be produced by stimulation of pulmonary and pleural tissue;[5] increased nasal and pharyngeal secretions may be produced by stimuli originating in either the lung or the upper gastrointestinal tract.[6] The oculocervical reflex which can be used beneficially in muscle energy osteopathic manipulative techniques has been implicated in the cervical vertigo symptomatology which occurs in cervical spondylosis, cervical inertial injuries (whiplash), cervical somatic dysfunction and cervical disk disease.

An understanding of the anatomy, physiology and pathophysiology of the head, neck and upper thoracic region is vital if the clinician is intent on providing optimum care for patients with EENT dysfunction.

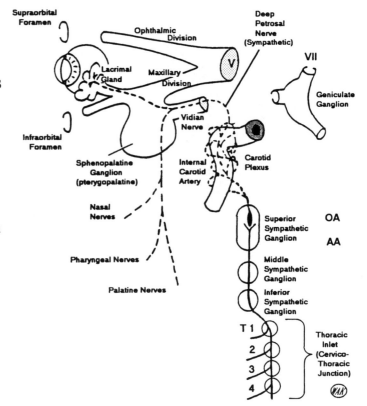

SYMPATHETICS:

EENT structures derive their sympathetic innervation from cell bodies located in spinal levels T1-4 with synapses between the pre-and post-ganglionic fibers occurring in the upper thoracic or cervical sympathetic ganglia. The sympathetic nerves generally follow the arterial supply to peripheral tissues.

2

Visceral afferent nerves, stimulated by organ dysfunction, often follow the same pathways as sympathetic innervation. Excessive input from a viscera of the head or neck produces facilitation of the upper thoracic cord segments and results in reflex stimulation of somatic tissues innervated by T1-4. The facilitated cord segment also encourages excessive sympathetic outflow from that segment to its associated viscera (T1-4, to the head and neck); it is also believed to be the basis for establishment of Chapman myofascial tender points related to visceral dysfunction.

Palpatory changes in the upper thoracic and cervical paraspinal tissues as well as traditional Chapman's reflex locations therefore indicate increased functional activity of the sympathetic nervous system in this region. On the other hand, physical findings such as Horner's syndrome[7] (constricted pupil, ptosis, and facial anhidrosis on the involved side) often indicate significant structural involvement or blockage of the sympathetic nervous system; this needs to be considered in the differential diagnostic process.

Increased sympathetic activity to the eye, ear, nose, and/or throat as well as the upper thoracic musculature augment the normal physiologic responses that those tissues are capable of providing. In general, the most common physiologic response is vasoconstriction leading to diminished nutrient supply to the tissues and reduced lymphatico-venous drainage. The body's ability to mount an immune response and to obtain effective concentrations of medications are reduced in areas of vasoconstriction and tissue congestion.

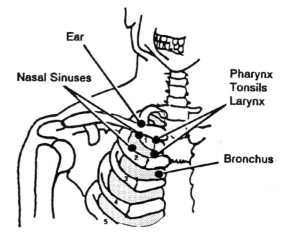

Chapman's Reflexes: Upper Respiratory Tract

Ear
Nasal Sinuses
Pharynx
Tonsils
Larynx
Bronchus

With chronic irritation, nasal and pharyngeal secretions from prolonged sympathetic stimulation of the respiratory epithelium becomes thick and sticky due to the increased number of goblet cells and decreased vascular elements. Sympathetic stimulation of the nasopharyngeal mucous membranes produces vasoconstriction, inhibits secretion, and results in dryness in several acute situations, including fever.[8] Often, dryness and cracking of the mucosa result in a breakdown of normal mucosal defense mechanisms and permits secondary bacterial infections to occur.

Dilation of the pupil (mydriasis) occurs with increased sympathetic activity to the eye; pupillary constriction results from a reduction or loss of sympathetic activity. Long term upper thoracic and cervical dysfunction with sympathicotonia have been implicated in the development of cloudiness of the lens.[9] In exophthalmic goiter, prolonged sympathetic activity producing contraction of the Mullerian orbital muscle combined with edema and lymphoid infiltration,[10] results in protrusion of the eyeball. Other eye phenomena in this same condition are due to hyperparasympathetic activity, such as the failure of the upper lid to follow the cornea when the eyes are lowered or a widening of the lid slits due to increased tone of the levator palpebrae muscle.

Sympathetic fibers innervate blood vessels which supply the thyroid and also innervate the cells which produce thyroid secretion. Increased local sympathetic activation, generalized adrenal activity or increased thyrotropic hormone from the anterior pituitary (any of these) increases thyroid glandular secretion.[11]

Common EENT signs and/or symptoms associated with increased sympathetic activity include photophobia, unsteadiness (slight vertigo), tinnitus, and thickened nasopharyngeal secretions. Hyperesthesia of the pharyngeal tissues usually makes patients anxious, causing them to "rasp, cough and expectorate to rid themselves of non-existing mucosities or some imaginary foreign body in the throat." Sweating is augmented and the patient may experience increased fatigue, palpitations, tachycardia, and insomnia. With mydriasis (a hyper-sympathetic event), narrow angle glaucoma may be made worse and intraocular pressures elevated.

While there are an abundance of symptoms produced by hypersympathetic activity, objective signs are difficult to measure with screening physical diagnostic tests. Palpatory changes as described earlier are accurate indicators and when present, warrant consideration in both the diagnostic and therapeutic arenas.

PARASYMPATHETICS:

Parasympathetic nerve fibers to the pupil are supplied by the third cranial nerve (oculomotor nerve). They synapse in the ciliary ganglia and then pass to the ciliary muscle where parasympathetic contraction of the pupil opposes sympathetic dilation. Contraction, from parasympathetic activity affecting the lens, shortens the eye's focal point. According to Pottenger, "When the excitability of the motor cells in the oculomotor nerve is very high, it may result in accommodation spasm."[12]

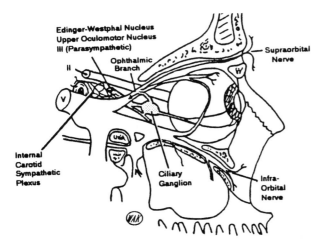

Parasympathetic nerve fibers to the lacrimal gland as well as to the nasopharyngeal mucosa travel via the seventh cranial nerve (facial). They synapse in the sphenopalatine ganglia. Parasympathetic hyper-activity is responsible for the production of tears from the lacrimal glands and profuse, clear, thin secretions from the mucosa of the nasopharynx and sinuses.

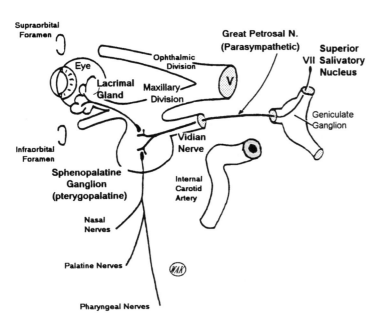

In the absence of histo-logical changes which may be produced by prolonged sympathicoto-nia, irritation of the nasopharyngeal mucosa results in a "runny nose" and watery eyes. A sphenopalatine syndrome is described as redness and "engorgement of the mucous membranes, photophobia, tearing and pain behind the eyeball, nose, neck, ear or temple."[13]

This syndrome is said to worsen cases of asthma due to lowered resistance of nasal mucosa to foreign protein and inadequate conditioning of the air entering the lungs.

Parasympathetic nerves to the thyroid arise from the superior and inferior laryngeal nerves and a branch from the main vagus nerve (cranial nerve X).

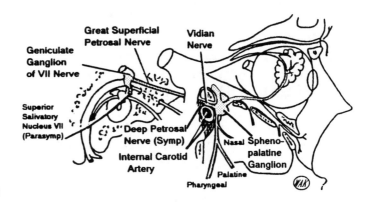

At this point its physiologic role in thyroid function is unknown; it is believed to be neither an activator nor an inhibitor of thyroid activity.

VENOUS AND LYMPHATIC SYSTEMS:

85% of the venous drainage from the head is accomplished via the jugular veins which pass through the right and left jugular foramina, formed in the occipitomastoid sutures between the occipital and the temporal bones. Venous congestion of the head leads to symptoms of cephalgia and anxiety.

The first sign of lymphatic congestion affecting EENT structures and attributable to fascial somatic dysfunction will appear as fullness in the supraclavicular tissues. The pre-auricular, post-auricular, tonsilar, submaxillary, submental, and posterior cervical lymph nodes should also be palpated for evidence of infection. Manipulative goals are directed toward opening lymphatic pathways while avoiding direct manipulation over swollen lymph nodes.

Lymphatic congestion leads to boggy, edematous tissues which are generally uncomfortable and which change local biochemical conditions and hinder homeostatic mechanisms. In nasopharyngeal dysfunction there will be diminished transport of nutrients to the tissues and a reduction in the movement of metabolic wastes from the mucosa. This hampers healing while increasing the possibilities of nasopharyngeal adhesions from repeated or serious infection.

Where the sclera, cornea, iris and ligamentum pectinatum meet is defined as the angle of the anterior chamber of the eye. "Upon the integrity of this angle depends the proper circulation of lymph to nourish the anterior portion of the eye";[14] glaucomatous changes have frequently been linked to poor lymphatic drainage of the eye.

In the inner ear, absorption of endolymph is believed to be important in the prevention of both endolymphatic hydrops ("glaucoma of the ear"[15]) and fibrosis of the endolymphatic duct which occurs in Meniere's disease. Meniere's disease is accompanied by symptoms of tinnitus, diminished hearing, and vertigo.

NEURAL SYSTEM:

A variety of EENT symptoms can be primarily explained by the effect of somatic dysfunction on motor or sensory nerves in the cranial and/or cervical regions. (Table 1, page 9)

A trauma history is important as EENT symptoms in a child or an adult often have their onset as a consequence of a difficult delivery or a trauma such as the inertial injury (whiplash) incurred in a motor vehicle accident. Dental trauma should also be a routine part of the historical questioning because of its propensity for creating cranial somatic dysfunction.

While the two most common pathophysiologic causes of extraocular muscle palsy are diabetes mellitus and aneurysm, extraocular muscle dysfunction is also a frequent sign of cranial somatic dysfunction and often responds well to osteopathic manipulative treatment directed at the attachments of the petrosphenoidal ligament. Because this ligament is formed by the anterior extensions of the fixed margins of the tentorum cerebelli to the body of the sphenoidal bone, treatment is typically directed to its attachments, particularly to the temporal and sphenoid bones.

Innervation to the extraocular muscles--cranial nerves III, IV and VI--is particularly vulnerable to dural stress as these nerves pass in close relationship to the petrosphenoidal ligament. Post-traumatically, symptoms of cranial nerve VI are the most common because this is the most vulnerable of the three nerves as it passes under the petrosphenoidal ligament.[16] Cranial nerve VI innervates the lateral rectus muscle so its dysfunction leads to medial strabismus. The effect of extraocular muscle dysfunction ranges from mild eye fatigue, headache and blurred or double vision to amblyopia, mild nystagmus, or strabismus. Any of these dysfunctions may respond favorably to OMT of the cranium.[17]

Other cranial nerves may be affected and lead to EENT symptoms. Dysfunction involving the olfactory nerve[18] (cranial nerve I) may lead to an altered sense of smell or to an impression of an odor that is not present. The trigeminal nerve (CN V) carries sensory information from many structures including the anterior and middle cranial fossae, the tentorum cerebelli, the mastoid air cells, the nasal mucosa, the cornea, and the temporomandibular joints. Dysfunction of the fifth cranial nerve may lead to headache[19] perceived in the anterior fossa, eyebrows, or sinuses; it is also considered in the differential diagnosis and treatment of trigeminal neuralgia (tic douloureux).[20] The buccal branch of cranial nerve V may be entrapped by trigger points[21] in the lateral pterygoid muscle and produce tingling in the cheek.

Dysfunction of cranial nerve VII is associated with complaint of a metallic taste or altered salivation. Finding somatic dysfunction in the cranium which could affect the facial nerve (CN VII) is also quite helpful in the differential diagnosis and treatment of Bell's palsy.[22] Vertigo, nystagmus and tinnitus are symptoms which may arise from involvement of the vestibulocochlear nerve (CN VIII).[23] With dysfunction of cranial nerves IX and X, infants may have poor suckling[24] or failure to thrive because of poor swallowing. Dysarthria may result from dysfunction of cranial nerve XII.

Palpation of the cranium for obvious strain patterns, occipital compression, and temporal malalignment is extremely helpful in ruling out cranial dysfunctional states which could lead to EENT symptoms. Treatment of any somatic dysfunction found is helpful in addressing the physiologic portion of the treatment protocol.

THE SOMATIC SYSTEM:

The myofascial system plays a significant role in EENT symptomatology. A number of myofascial trigger points (TPs) have been well documented by Travell and Simons that refer pain to, and/or cause dysfunction of, the eye, ear, nose, Eustachian tube, and throat. Specific questions relating to the activation of the pertinent muscles outlined in Table 1 (page 9) should therefore be posed. All myofascial trigger points and particularly those in the head and neck region, are aggravated by cold and emotional stress. In this area, emotional stress symptoms[25] such as bruxism and clenching of the teeth are particularly pertinent as they produce TPs in the masseter and pterygoid muscles. Frowning or squinting sets up TPs[26] in the orbicularis oculi and occipitalis muscles. These muscles are also activated by excessive gum chewing, worn teeth or dentures, occlusal disharmony, TMJ, and prolonged dental procedures.

Symptoms referred by myofascial dysfunction to the eye are most prominently seen with TPs in the sternal division of the sternocleidomastoid muscle.[27] Motor vehicle accidents, especially those from the rear[28] when the head is turned, frequently cause trigger points in the sternocleidomastoid, splenius cervicis, and trapezius muscles. Postural disorders must be ruled out[29] as a perpetuating factor in those cases where the trigger points are difficult to eradicate.

Because of ipsilateral visual disturbances including blurring, diminution of perceived light and apparent ptosis from spasm of the orbicularis oculi in the reference zone, the patient may report a need to tip the head backwards to look up. TPs in the obicularis oculi muscle will also cause excess ipsilateral lacrimation and conjunctival reddening due to vascular engorgement.[30] TPs in the orbicularis oculi muscle may result in patient complaints of "jumpy print" while reading.[31] Splenius cervicis TPs[32] will produce ipsilateral blurring of near vision without conjunctivitis or dizziness as well as pain in the eye and orbit. Those in the occipitalis muscle refer pain behind the eye and in the eyeball and eyelid while those in the trapezius might refer pain to the back of the orbit.

The underlying cause of functional ear symptoms should be carefully and systematically sorted out. The role of cranial nerve dysfunction and lymphatic congestion has already been discussed with regard to tinnitus, vertigo, and/or hearing disorders. Cranial somatic dysfunction is a frequent cause of functional symptoms. External rotation of the temporal bone is associated with low-pitched roaring tinnitus; fixed internal rotation associated with high-pitched tinnitus; and both potentially causing vertigo.[33]

TABLE 1: TRAVELL TRIGGERS WITH EENT SYMPTOMS;

EYE SYMPTOMS AND/OR PAIN:

> Sternal Division of Sternocleidomastoid Muscle
> Splenius Cervicis Muscle
> Occipitalis Muscle
> Orbicularis Oculi Muscle
> Trapezius Muscle

EAR PAIN, TINNITUS, AND/OR DIMINISHED HEARING:

> Deep Portion of Masseter Muscle
> Clavicular Portion of Sternocleidomastoid Muscle
> Medial Pterygoid Muscle
> Occipitalis Muscle (Possible)

EUSTACHIAN TUBE DYSFUNCTION:

> Medial Pterygoid Muscle

NOSE PAIN:

> Orbicularis Oculi Muscle

MAXILLARY SINUS PAIN AND/OR SINUS SYMPTOMS:

> Lateral Pterygoid Muscle
> Masseter Muscle
> Sternal Division of Sternocleidomastoid Muscle

THROAT PAIN AND/OR PAIN OR DIFFICULTY SWALLOWING:

> Medial Pterygoid Muscle
> Digastric Muscle

CRANIAL NERVE ENTRAPMENT:

> V_A (Buccal Nerve Branch): Lateral Pterygoid Muscle
> XI : Sternocleidomastoid Muscle

Otalgia can be referred[34] from teeth, tongue, tonsils, esophagus, TMJ and from cervical/cranial somatic dysfunction through cranial nerves V, IX and X or C1-2. To these factors can be added Eustachian tube dysfunction and myofascial trigger points.

Both secretory and acute otitis media often arise from Eustachian tube dysfunction. The middle ear is normally ventilated 3-4 times per minute as the Eustachian tube opens during swallowing, sneezing or yawning. Even mild infection can cause mucosal swelling sufficient to block the Eustachian tube[35] leading to pressure changes within the middle ear, retraction of the tympanic membrane, serous otitis and hearing loss. Under these conditions oxygen is absorbed through the blood vessels in the mucous membrane of the middle ear. In the pathogenesis of secretory otitis media, a relative negative pressure develops with Eustachian tube dysfunction leading to mild retraction of the tympanic membrane. This can be demonstrated on physical examination by abnormal light reflection on the tympanic membrane and by poor insufflation. The negative middle ear pressure causes a transudate from the blood vessels of the mucous membrane of the middle ear. This produces an amber to gray colored appearance to the tympanic membrane, a fluid level and bubbles may be seen on otologic examination. A conductive hearing deficit develops in patients with secretory otitis and it may last for months.

Stein's textbook, Internal Medicine, states that the most important predisposing factor in developing acute otitis media is an acute nasopharyngeal infection, usually viral, causing Eustachian tube dysfunction that allows microbial proliferation and infection in the middle ear, especially when combined with other inadequate host factors.[36] Cranial somatic dysfunction has also proven to be a predisposing factor for recurrent pediatric otitis media.[37]

Eustachian tube dysfunction may occur from tissue swelling, edema, and/or adhesions forming after tonsillectomy or after repeated or serious infections. It may also arise from trigger points in the medial pterygoid[38] muscle or from dysfunction of cranial nerve X. Additionally, it has been associated with cranial somatic dysfunction[39]--especially internal rotation of the temporal bone or torsion or sidebending-rotation of the sphenobasilar symphysis. Regardless of the etiology, Eustachian tube dysfunction has been associated with a variety of patient signs, symptoms, or disorders including diminished hearing, pain with altitude changes, tinnitus, recurrent infections, secretory and acute otitis media, asymmetrical elevation of the uvula upon phonation, and vertigo. Because any of these symptoms may arise from Eustachian tube dysfunction, physical examination of the posterior pharynx, palpation of the medial pterygoid muscle and cranium, and visualization with insufflation of the tympanic membrane should be performed.

TABLE 2: SELECTED DIFFERENTIAL POINTS IN DIAGNOSES ASSOCIATED WITH FUNCTIONAL EAR COMPONENTS

DIAGNOSIS	EAR SENSATION	TINNITUS	DECREASED HEARING	VERTIGO/ DIZZINESS
Meniere's Disease	Fullness	85-90% Unilateral	85-95% Unilateral 10-15% Bilateral	Vertigo
Hypothyroidism	(-)	(-)	Bilateral	Dizzy
Hyperthyroidism	(-)	Bilateral	(-)	lightheadedness
Eustachian Dysfunction	Fullness	(+) Unilateral	Conductive Unilaterally	(?)
Labyrinthitis	(+/-)	(-)	(+)	Dizzy
Temporal Bone Somatic Dysfunction	with OA or vagal involv.	(+/-) Unilateral	(+/-)	Dizzy or Vertigo
TP Deep Masseter	Deep Pain	Unilateral	(-)	(-)
TP Clavicular Portion of Sternocleidomastoid	(+/-)	(-)	Unilateral	Contributes to Carsickness Seasickness
TP Medial Pterygoid	Stuffiness	(-)	(-)	(-)
TP Occipitalis	Ache	(-)	slightly	(-)
Post-Concussion Syndrome	(-)	(+/-)	Sensorineural	Vertigo
Salicylate Toxicity	(-)	Bilateral	(-)	(-)

Other ear symptoms attributable to myofascial trigger points (TPs) include those in the deep portion of the masseter, the clavicular portion of the sternocleidomastoid (SCM), the medial pterygoid, and according to Kellgren, the occipitalis muscle. Variables in the presentation of these points and other differentials are detailed in Table 2 on page 11.

The low roaring tinnitus experienced in TPs from the deep portion of the masseter[40] muscle will often vary when the jaw is opened wide. The stuffiness in the ear caused by TPs in the medial pterygoid[41] muscle is felt to be due to Eustachian tube dysfunction which arises from inability of the tensor veli palatini muscle to move the medial pterygoid and associated fascia aside to open that structure. Not included in Table 2, are the TPs of the trapezius[42] which includes among its many other referral sites, the postauricular area.

Sinus symptoms can also arise from myofascial structures. TPs in the lateral pterygoid[43] muscle refer severe pain to the maxillary region as well as autonomically stimulating excessive secretions from the maxillary sinuses. Pain referred from this TP and from TPs in the superficial upper portion of the masseter muscle give rise to complaints of "sinus attack" and often result in incorrect and therefore ineffective treatment for sinusitis. Dysfunctional TPs in the sternal division of the sternocleidomastoid[44] cause coryza and maxillary sinus congestion. Nose pain, per se, is rarely caused by TPs other than those in the orbicularis oculi[45] muscle.

Throat pain arises from myofascial triggers in either the medial pterygoid[46] and digastric[47] muscles. Swallowing is painful with the former and difficult with the latter.

III. TREATMENT

After a thorough diagnostic evaluation, a tentative diagnosis is made. Formation of a rational osteopathic treatment for this initial diagnosis must:

o .. consider the patient's body as a unit
o .. support structure and functional components
o .. support and enhance the homeostatic mechanisms involved

The most effective treatment plan is directed at the cause of the complaints and not at the symptoms.

In general, this section will consider primarily the manipulative techniques which fulfill the objectives mentioned in the previous paragraph. Treatment of the upper thoracic and cervical regions effectively addresses the sympathetic component. Lymphatic congestion is best accomplished by first opening the pathways--especially the thoracic inlet and anterior and posterior cervical soft tissues--and then enhancing the fluid movement with diaphragmatic techniques, lymph pumps and effleurage. Treatment of the parasympathetic component, when it is present, often involves use of manipulative techniques to the cranium and/or occipitocervical junction. In certain circumstances, specific manipulative techniques, exercises or dietary considerations may be applied to the general treatment plan outlined above.

THE EYE:

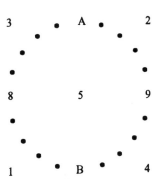

Effleurage over the eyelid and globe is often beneficial with edema of the eyelid and scleral edema. Avoid stroking over the lid when the patient is wearing contacts or if any other ophthalmic foreign body is suspected.

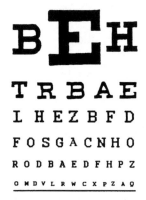

Some patients have an impaired ability to focus their eyes and, whether near- or far-sighted, may benefit from a series of eye exercises developed by H.A. Richardson, D.O.[48]

Using an enlarged chart like the one illustrated above, this is one of six eye exercises that Dr. Richardson had his patients perform.

"To be effective the patient must be motivated enough to perform the exercises regularly. Pin a large "AB" test chart on the wall with the figure 5 on a direct line with the end of your nose. Stand three inches away and see that your nose is on a direct line with the figure 5. Now look at No. 1, then at No. 2, then back to No. 1. Do this five times, stretching the muscles of the eyes each time. Then shift from No. 3 to No. 4, five times each way. Do not move the head. Then shift from No. 8 to No. 9 five times each way. Then look up at A and down at B five times up and down. Then while you remain the same distance from the chart, starting at A, shift the eyes from one dot to the other all the way around the circle back to A. Do this five times to the right, then five times to the left. Blink each time that you look at a dot; but do not move your head when exercising. Now close the eyes tightly five times. Then look at No. 5 and close the eyes for a second; then open them and look at No. 5 again. Open and close them five times, looking at No. 5 again. Open and close them five times, looking at No. 5 each time. This exercises both the internal and external rectus muscles at the same time. Now close your eyes and cover them with the palms of the hands, being sure to exclude all light and relax in this position for five minutes. If one eye is weaker than the other, you should cover the stronger eye and do more exercising with the weaker eye. Now take your seat at about ten feet from the "AB" test chart and read all of the letters on the card, shifting the eyes rapidly from the bottom to the top of each letter, blinking every time you shift the eyes.

After you have read all of the letters on the card at least once, you should again cover the eyes with the palms of the hands and relax for a few minutes being careful not to put any pressure on the eyeballs."[49]

T.J. Ruddy, D.O.,[50] an osteopathic ophthalmologist, also developed a series of muscle energy techniques designed to balance extra-ocular muscle tone. These techniques utilize traditional muscle energy principles with the physician applying resistance against the ocular globe as the patient attempts to look in a specific direction. This form of OMT, combined with cranial techniques to improve the structure-function relationship of extraocular muscle innervation, has been helpful in patients with functional diplopia, strabismus, cephalgia secondary to eye strain, amblyopia, and other conditions in which somatic dysfunction of the extraocular muscles plays a role.

Another technique applied directly to the globe has been utilized for patients with mild chronic glaucoma.[51] The purpose of this technique is to improve fluid drainage and constitutes part of a total treatment program. With the patient's eyes closed, the physician places a finger across the eyelid from lateral to medial. With a finger of the other hand, a light percussion is performed over finger that lies on the closed eyelid. In one study, intraocular tension averaged 3-5 mm Hg reduction 60 minutes after an OMT regimen.[52] In a double blind, randomized study of intraocular pressure of normal and chronic, open angle glaucoma patients, significant pressure changes were also seen 6 to 60 minutes after osteopathic manipulative treatment.[53] Acute closed-angle glaucoma, on the other hand, is an ocular emergency which may produce blindness in 3-5 days unless treated medically.

Where structural problems such as entropion or extropion lead to functional disorders such as poor drainage of tears through the nasolacrimal system or chronic recurrent pathophysiology such as the inflammation seen in chronic conjunctivitis, the best treatment is probably surgical repair of the structural disorder. However, where functional problems lead to eye pain, blurred vision or reddening, manipulative or spray-and-stretch techniques should be applied to specific trigger muscles. (See Table I, page 9.)

THE EAR:

In patients with significant cranial somatic dysfunction who are also experiencing vertigo or tinnitus, a therapeutic trial of manipulation is warranted. Goals include achieving a balance between the temporal bones, normalizing the cranial rhythmic impulse, and removing areas of dural strain. In addition, each of the muscles listed in Table 2 page 11 that meet the patient's presentation should be palpated and treated if a myofascial trigger is found.

Patients with structural adhesions affecting the Eustachian tube may complain of deafness, otalgia with altitude changes, recurrent otitis media, vertigo and/or tinnitis. They may benefit from lysis of these nasopharyngeal adhesions. A technique, referred to as "finger surgery", was popularized by C.H. Muncie, M.D.[54] It is often effective in modifying the structure sufficiently to restore normal Eustachian tube function.

Yawning and swallowing are essential to normal Eustachian tube function, therefore dysfunction affecting cranial nerves IX, or V, or any of the myofascial structures involved in these actions can compromise maximal Eustachian tube function. Myofascial dysfunction in the medial pterygoid muscles and those attached to the hyoid bone are particularly likely to disturb the opening of the Eustachian tube. These dysfunctions respond well to OMT.

The frequency of pediatric otitis media is increased in relation to a number of somatic factors (number of cranial strain patterns,[55] presence of plagiocephaly, or Eustachian tube dysfunction[56]), environmental factors (exposure to tobacco smoking[57] and woodheating,[58] or participation in day care), and familial factors (history of sibling or parental otitis media).[59]

The treatment of choice for acute otitis media would address the underlying Eustachian tube dysfunction, provide antibiotics capable of managing both *Strept pneumonia* and *Hemophilus influenza*[60] and support host elements. Such a regimen permits the body's homeostatic elements the best opportunity to interrupt the natural progress of the disease, spontaneous perforation of the tympanic membrane with closure and return of hearing in 1-2 weeks. Because secretory otitis media has a sterile effusion, antibiotics are not helpful unless it is associated with a bacterial rhinitis, sinusitis, or nasopharyngitis. Pseudoephedrine for vasoconstriction may be of some symptomatic relief, but the osteopathic physician should go back and treat any underlying nasopharyngeal structural or functional condition which may be causing the Eustachian tube dysfunction. Antihistamines may only be appropriate when allergic factors are associated with Eustachian tube dysfunction.

Manipulative treatment in Meniere's disease has been specifically described as "beneficial."[61] One study of OMT in Meniere's patients revealed excellent results or significant improvement in 79% of cases.[62] OMT addressing dural restrictions, and especially those associated with temporal bone dysfunction,[63] is particularly helpful in our experience as are diagnosis and treatment of the lymphatic and autonomic components.

THE NOSE AND SINUSES:

W. Hadley Hoyt III, D.O. in his article, "Current concepts in management of sinus disease,"[64] states, "OMT should be included in the treatment of sinusitis." He notes that OMT should address parasympathetic and sympathetic fibers as homeostasis of their autonomic functions may prevent ostial occlusion. Sensory fibers to the sinuses (originating in the trigeminal nerve) should also be addressed.

Stimulation of the sphenopalatine ganglia[65] results in a brief period in which there is production of profuse, thin nasal secretions, a parasympathetic response. This may prove helpful in the symptomatic relief of patients with sinusitis or patients whose thick nasal secretions have been difficult to clear from the nasal passageways. The pressure applied to the site needed to affect the sphenopalatine ganglion will elicit "exquisite" tenderness if active lateral pterygoid myofascial trigger points are present.[66] Often the referred maxillary sinus pain and autonomically induced excessive secretions will resolve with the inhibition that occurs with this technique.[67] Research utilizing rhinomanometry has shown that following osteopathic manipulative treatment there is a reduction in the amount of work required by the nose during breathing.[68]

Manipulative techniques to free somatic dysfunction in the cranium[69] (especially the frontal-ethmoidal and facial bones) or to improve the pumping motion through the vomer are beneficial for improved nasal sinus function. They are extremely helpful in patients with dysfunctional, allergic, or infectious etiologies for rhinitis, acute sinusitis, or the pharyngitis resulting from post-nasal drainage. CV4 cranial technique is felt to act through fluid mobilization and increased pump potency; regardless of mechanism, shortly after applying this technique, most patients note significant clearing of the sinuses.

Treatment to normalize the body's response to sensory input along branches of the trigeminal is helpful in reducing reflex symptoms ranging from sinus headache to sneezing. This may be accomplished with gentle rotatory stimulation over the bony foramina of the supraorbital and infraorbital nerves. (See the next section entitled "Osteopathic Considerations in the Common Cold.")

In patients with structural abnormalities such as nasal septal deformity or chronic sinusitis, surgery becomes the osteopathic treatment of choice.[70] When functional and otherwise transient changes in acute sinusitis are inadequately treated, irreversible structural changes may result. Thus, in chronic sinusitis, when the normal ciliated epithelium is replaced with stratified squamous cells incapable of homeostatic clearance mechanisms,[71] antibiotic and manipulative therapy is rendered ineffective. Hoyt notes, "Functional sinus surgery offers new hope to the patient who has failed to respond to conservative osteopathic medical treatment"[72] and can relieve associated somatic cephalgic manifestations.

THE THROAT:

The techniques described previously for the Eustachian tube and sphenopalatine ganglia are also indicated to treat dysfunctions of the pharynx. Soft tissue techniques to the anterior cervical fascia and gentle manipulation to correct any hyoid dysfunction are also extremely beneficial in reestablishing normal function in this region and permits the patient significant symptomatic relief.

Addressing the anterior cervical fascias and hyoid bone is frequently helpful in thyroid dysfunction, but because this is an endocrine gland and under the control of the pituitary, evaluation and treatment of any cranial dysfunction[73] should also be performed.

THE ENT UNIT:

Mandibular drainage technique is effective in encouraging drainage from the nasopharyngeal area and opening the Eustachian tube. It is therefore helpful in decongestion of a large part of the ENT unit.

The procedure is described by Angus Cathie, D.O. (after Galbreath) in his discussion of the sinobronchial syndrome[74] and is also mentioned by Harold I. Magoun, D.O.[75] The patient is treated in the supine position with a slight elevation of the head which is rotated 90^{0} to the non-involved side. The operator stabilizes the frontoparietal region with one hand and places his/her fingers of the other hand below the zygomatic arch and over the TMJ with the heel near the symphysis menti. The patient is instructed to relax his/her jaw while the operator applies a slow, firm pressure downward, forward, and medial. This is released and repeated alternately to apply a "make/break tension" to the pterygoid muscles. This decongests the rich pterygoid venous plexus which drains the tissues noted above. Relaxation of the medial pterygoid muscle also enables the tensor veli palatini muscle to functionally open the Eustachian tube.

While usually utilized to facilitate diagnosis, treatment of ENT Chapman's points with generalized soft tissue techniques or specific rotatory stimulation can be postulated to beneficially modify sympathetic outflow. It is noted that symptomatic relief is afforded the upper respiratory tract when these reflex points are treated as a system. For comfort and practicality, the posterior points are treated first and the anterior points may be gently treated if they remain.

↑ CRI → ↑ Endolymphatic Flow
Oculocervical - Muscle Energy
Cervicals C3-5 (Phrenic Nerve)
T1-12 and Ribs 1-12 (Somatic Nerves and Respiration)
Thoracolumbar Junction (Diaphragm Attachment)
Medial pterygoid muscle
Hyoid Soft Tissue for Eustachian Tube

```
┌──────────────────────────┐
│ Somatic Dysfunction      │
│   ┌──────────────┐       │
│   │ facil. seg.  │       │
│   └──────────────┘       │
│     Sympathetics ────────┼──────────── Parasympathetics
└──────────────────────────┘
```

Rib Raising
  T1-4
Cervical Fascias
  (Cerv. Ganglia)   TREATMENT PLAN FOR   Sphenopalatine
Chapman's Reflexes   EENT DYSFUNCTION   Ganglion Technique,
Eye: Cranial OMT to Affect
  T1-2   Cranial Nerves
  Ciliospinal Center   Lymphatics   (Cranial N-VII)

Thoracic Inlets
Abdominal Diaphragm
Effleurage
Lymphatic Pumps
Ruddy's Resistive Duction
  Ocular - Muscle Energy
Stroking (Ocular)

SYMPATHETIC EFFECTS

↑ Tone:

  ↑ Vasoconstriction
  ↑ Thickens Secretions (↑ Number of Goblet Cells)
  ↓ Drainage
  Mydriasis → Worsening of Glaucoma

LYMPHATIC EFFECTS

Impaired Lymph Flow:

  ↓ Drainage
  ↑ Congestion
  ↑ Endolymphatic Pressure → Possible Fibrosis of
                             Endolymphatic Channel
                             With Stasis
                                  ↓
                           → Meniere's Disease

PARASYMPATHETIC EFFECTS

↑ Tone:

  ↑ Thinning of Secretions
  Improved Drainage

IV. SUMMARY

Reflex mechanisms are extremely active in integrated EENT functions. Somatic dysfunction modifies normal reflex activities and may produce dysfunctional states whose symptoms must be differentiated as to whether they are functional (somatic dysfunction) or pathological. In disease situations, somatic dysfunction reduces the efficacy of the body's homeostatic mechanism. Successful manipulation of somatic dysfunction constitutes either a therapeutic trial or an important support to homeostasis. Its incorporation into the treatment program speeds healing and decreases morbidity while simultaneously providing symptomatic relief for the patient.

ADDITIONAL EENT BIBLIOGRAPHY:

Norfolk DF: Cranial nerve syndromes: relationship to musculoskeletal lesions of the cervical spine. The Journal of Osteopathy 1962; 69(8): 17-22.

Gayral L, Neuwirth E: Oto-neuro-ophalmologic manifestations of cervical origin. New York State J Med 1954; 54: 1920-1922.

REFERENCES:

1. Magoun HI: Osteopathy in the Cranial Field. Kirksville, Journal Printing Co, 3rd ed, 1976, p 276.
2. Pottenger FM Symptoms of Visceral Disease. St Louis, CV Mosby Co, 7th ed, 1953. pp 239-40, 374-391.
3. Op cit p 381.
4. Travell JG, Simons DG Myofascial Pain and Dysfunction: The Trigger Point Manual. Baltimore, Williams and Wilkins, 1983, p 209.
5. Pottenger FM Symptoms of Visceral Disease. St Louis, CV Mosby Co, 7th ed, 1953, p 239.
6. Op cit pp 239-240, 378.
7. Stein JH (ed) Internal Medicine. Boston, Little, Brown & Co, 3rd ed, 1990, p 1897.
8. Pottenger FM Symptoms of Visceral Disease. St Louis, CV Mosby Co, 7th ed, 1953, pp 377-8.
9. Cole WV: Experimental evidence, in Hoag JM (ed) Osteopathic Medicine. New York, MᶜGraw-Hill, 1969, ch 8, p 119.
10. Pottenger FM Symptoms of Visceral Disease. St Louis, CV Mosby Co, 7th ed, 1953, pp 384-6.
11. Cole WV: Experimental evidence, in Hoag JM (ed) Osteopathic Medicine. New York, McGraw-Hill, 1969, ch 8, p 119.
12. Pottenger FM Symptoms of Visceral Disease. St Louis, CV Mosby Co, 7th ed, 1953, p 385.
13. Magoun HW: Neuroscience studies in Goldstein M (ed) The Research Status of Spinal Manipulative Therapy, Bethesda MD, US Department of

Health, Education and Welfare (NINCDS Monograph #15), 1975, pp 213-6.

14. Wolf AH: Osteopathic manipulation in eye, ear, nose, and throat disease. AAO Yearbook 1962: 133-40

15. Gibson WPR: The diagnosis and treatment of Meniere's disease. The Practitioner 1978; 221: 718-722.

16. Magoun HI Osteopathy in the Cranial Field. Kirksville, Journal Printing Company, 3rd ed, 1976, p 293.

17. Op cit pp 267,284, 293.

18. Op cit p 167.

19. Op cit pp 76, 185, 290.

20. Op cit pp 294-300.

21. Travell JG, Simons DG Myofascial Pain and Dysfunction: A Trigger Point Manual. Baltimore, Williams & Wilkins, 1983, p 266.

22. Magoun HI Osteopathy in the Cranial Field. Kirksville, Journal Printing Company, 3rd ed, 1976, p 269.

23. Op cit p 150.

24. Op cit p 234.

25. Travell JG, Simons DG Myofascial Pain and Dysfunction: A Trigger Point Manual. Baltimore, Williams & Wilkins, 1983, pp 219, 249.

26. Op cit pp 285, 293.

27. Op cit p 203.

28. Op cit p 299.

29. Op cit pp 103-114.

30. Op cit p 203.

31. Op cit pp 296, 298.

32. Op cit pp 285, 288.

33. Magoun HI Osteopathy in the Cranial Field. Kirksville, Journal Printing Company, 3rd ed, 1976, pp 151, 215.

34. Op cit p 286.

35. Moore KL Clinically Oriented Anatomy. Baltimore, Williams & Wilkins, 2nd ed, 1985, p 970.

36. Stein JH Internal Medicine. Boston, Little, Brown, & Co, 3rd ed, 1990, p 1262.

37. Degenhardt BD, Kuchera ML: The prevalence of cranial dysfunction in children with a history of otitis media from kindergarten to third grade. Mead-Johnson Fellowship Paper, 1993.

38. Travell JG, Simons DG Myofascial Pain and Dysfunction: A Trigger Point Manual. Baltimore, Williams & Wilkins, 1983, p 249.

39. Magoun HI Osteopathy in the Cranial Field. Kirksville, Journal Printing Company, 3rd ed, 1976, pp 151, 215.

40. Op cit p 221.

41. Op cit p 249.

42. Op cit p 184.

43. Op cit pp 263-4.

44. Op cit p 203.

45. Op cit p 282.

46. Op cit p 252.

47. Op cit p 276.

48. Richardson RA <u>Increasing The Strength Of The Eyes and the Eye Muscles Without the Aid of Glasses</u>. Kansas City, The Eyesight and Health Association, 1925.
49. Op cit pp 52-53.
50. Ruddy TJ: Osteopathic manipulation in eye, ear, nose, and throat disease. <u>AAO Yearbook</u> 1962: pp 133-40.
51. Ibid
52. Misischia PJ: The evaluation of intraocular tension following osteopathic manipulation. <u>JAOA</u> July 1981, 80:750.
53. Feely RA, Castillo TA, Greiner JV. Osteopathic manipulative treatment and intraocular pressure. <u>JAOA</u> Sept 82, 82:60.
54. Muncie CH <u>Prevention and Cure of Deafness Through Muncie Reconstructive Method</u>. 1960.
55. Degenhardt BD, Kuchera ML: The prevalence of cranial dysfunction in children with a history of otitis media from kindergarten to third grade. Mead-Johnson Fellowship Paper, 1993.
56. Stein HJ <u>Internal Medicine</u>. Boston, Little, Brown & Co, 3rd ed, 1990, p 1262.
57. Hinton AE: Surgery for otitis media with effusion in children and its relationship to parental smoking. <u>J Laryngol Otol</u> 103: 550, 1989.
58. Degenhardt BD, Kuchera ML: The prevalence of cranial dysfunction in children with a history of otitis media from kindergarten to third grade. Mead-Johnson Fellowship Paper, 1993.
59. Degenhardt BD, Kuchera ML: The prevalence of cranial dysfunction in children with a history of otitis media from kindergarten to third grade. Mead-Johnson Fellowship Paper, 1993.
60. Stein HJ <u>Internal Medicine</u>. Boston, Little, Brown & Co, 3rd ed, 1990, p 1262.
61. Cole WV: Disorders of the nervous system, in Hoag JM (ed) <u>Osteopathic Medicine</u>. New York, McGraw-Hill, 1969, ch 20, p 315.
62. Korr IM (ed) <u>The Neurobiologic Mechanisms in Manipulative Therapy</u>. New York, Plenum Press, 1977, p 61.
63. Magoun HI <u>Osteopathy in the Cranial Field</u>. Kirksville, Journal Printing Co, 3rd ed, 1976, p 281.
64. Hoyt (III) WH: Current concepts in management of sinus disease. <u>JAOA</u> October 1990; 90(10); pp 913-919.
65. Op cit p 183.
66. Travell JG, Simons DG <u>Myofascial Pain and Dysfunction: A Trigger Point Manual</u>. Baltimore, Williams & Wilkins, 1983, p 265.
67. Op cit p 263.
68. Kaluza, Sherbin M: "The physiologic response of the nose to osteopathic manipulative treatment: Preliminary report." <u>JAOA</u> May 83, 82:654-60
69. Magoun HI <u>Osteopathy in the Cranial Field</u>. Kirksville, Journal Printing Co, 3rd ed, 1976, pp 289-291.
70. Rebik JM, McIntire LD, Hoyt WH (III), McIntire KD: Ethmoid sinus disease and nasal septal deformities as etiologies of chronic cephalgia: Results of surgical management. <u>JAOA</u> (October 1990): 897-907.
71. Stein HJ <u>Internal Medicine</u>. Boston, Little, Brown & Co, 3rd ed, 1990, p 1262.
72. Hoyt (III) WH: Current concepts in management of sinus disease. <u>JAOA</u> October 1990; 90(10); p 918.

73. Magoun HI <u>Osteopathy in the Cranial Field</u>. Kirksville, Journal Printing Co, 3rd ed, 1976, p 214.
74. Cathie A: Sino-bronchial syndrome. <u>AAO Yearbook</u>, 1974: 180-1.
75. Magoun HI <u>Osteopathy in the Cranial Field</u>. Kirksville, Journal Printing Co, 3rd ed, 1976, p 215.

OSTEOPATHIC CONSIDERATIONS IN THE COMMON COLD AND OTHER UPPER RESPIRATORY INFECTIONS

I. INTRODUCTION

Probably no disease causes so much aggravation to so many people as the common cold. Its viral etiology makes treatment with antibiotics ineffective; in fact, studies indicate that the use of antibiotics in a viral infection only prolongs the symptomatic stage of the infection. Modern medical treatment consists of symptomatic care with a polypharmacy that often includes antihistamines, analgesics and decongestants administered by spray, tablets or capsules. This is a less than optimum protocol.

The common cold affects the function of the upper respiratory tract--nasal passages, sinuses, ears, pharynx and bronchial tubes. The nasal passages are a very small part of the total human anatomy but they have a very important role in the maintenance of health. Though they are only 4 inches in length from the nares to the posterior pharynx, air from a single inhalation travels that distance in 1/4 second, is warmed to 96.8 degrees, 75% humidified, and practically filtered clean regardless of the condition of the air outside the body.

A special type of respiratory epithelium, composed of a combination of ciliated columnar and goblet cells, provides the means of effectively filtering and moisturizing the air. In a state of health, the epithelial ratio of goblet to ciliated cells is maintained by a predominant influence from its parasympathetic innervation. The resulting secretion is present in two layers and normally the layer of mucus next to the cells is clear with a saliva-like consistency.

Inhaled air is warmed and humidified by the structural nature of three nasal turbinates which line each nasal passage. These turbinates increase the surface area to which inhaled air is exposed and dilation of their abundant thin-walled blood vessels effectively warms the air, even in a very cold external environment.

Because of their shape and location, the turbulence of the inhaled air is increased so that foreign particles are thrown against the fluent but sticky superficial layer of the mucous blanket. Foreign particles stick to this superficial layer where lysozyme, an enzyme present in this mucus, kills virus and bacteria on contact. Both layers of the entire mucous blanket are moved slowly toward the back of the pharynx by the action of the ciliated cells as their cilia move the deeper saliva-like layer of mucus.

Mucus that arrives at the posterior pharynx is usually swallowed. The mucous blanket is completely replaced 3-4 times in every 24 hour period, amounting to a normal total production of 1.5 pints of mucus per day. Any bacteria or virus remaining alive after being swallowed will be killed by the gastric acid in the stomach.

The constant movement of air through the nasal passages would dry out the mucous membranes without homeostatic mechanisms. In order to protect the mucosal blanket and the nasal epithelium from drying out, 80% of the normal population have "nasal cycles." These are alternating patency cycles of the nasal passages during which one naris assumes the dominant role of air passage while the other one "rests". When working properly, this fluctuation is not noticed because the total air resistance is unchanged. If one or both nares are unable to dilate because of allergic congestion, infection, or some structural problem such as nasal deviation or a fractured nose, the total resistance to the air passing through the nasal passages is greatly increased. Patients with any of these conditions interpret the usual resting stage of the nasal cycle as "nasal congestion".

It is important to remember that the same stratified ciliated columnar epithelium which lines the nasal passages also lines the sinuses and the bronchial tubes. (Stratified squamous epithelium in the respiratory tract is found only in the posterior pharynx.)

II. PATHOPHYSIOLOGY

Infection begins with decreased resistance of the host. A person can often recall many etiological stressful situations which can reduce resistance of the body. Initially there appears to be increased parasympathetic activity and the mucus becomes more profuse and watery. The common cold viruses, such as the rhinovirus, do not attack the epithelial cell walls but produce inflammation with increased transudation of fluids rich in kinins (bradykinins, lysylbradykinin). These set up the symptoms of inflammation and predispose to bacterial infection. Perhaps the body is trying to functionally flush out or dilute the pathogen or irritant. As the viral invasion becomes more advanced, visceral afferent impulses to the spinal cord increase. Most visceral afferent nerves share the fascial pathways traveled by the sympathetic nerves which innervate that organ, so these impulses arrive at the same cord levels as that organ's sympathetic innervation. Afferent impulses from the sinuses and other head structures synapse in the dorsal horns of spinal cord segments T1-4 and those from the bronchial tree feed into the spinal cord at the T1-6 levels.

Reduction in the natural resistance of the body to protect and defend the air passages allows secondary bacterial infection to occur and in the case of the influenza virus, a direct attack upon the cell wall of the respiratory epithelium. Influenza virus invades the epithelial cells to use the cells' own metabolic processes in the production of more viruses. The fate of the infected cells depends upon how severely the virus disturbs the cells' metabolism. There may be local congestion, mucosal ulceration, sloughing, and exudate formation. Exudate makes an excellent media for bacterial growth and bacteria in the region take advantage of the denuded surfaces and "protein rich cellular broth." Secondary infection by *Haemophilus influenza* and *Staphlococcus pyogens* bacteria is common.

A steady stream of visceral afferent impulses from a dysfunctional upper respiratory tract "facilitates" the upper four to six thoracic spinal cord segments and permits viscerovisceral reflexes that result in excessive sympathetic output to the respiratory epithelium of the head, neck and bronchial tubes. In the common cold, palpatory evidence of tenderness and spasticity may be evident from the cervical through the thoracolumbar junction, but especially from C1 to T3.[1]

Presynaptic sympathetic fibers destined for the head and neck synapse in the cervical sympathetic ganglia while those destined for the lungs and the bronchial epithelium synapse in the T1-6 paraspinal chain ganglia. Postsynaptic sympathetic fibers travel through the respiratory plexus to the bronchial epithelium of the lungs or through the carotid plexus, the deep petrosal nerve, the nerve of the pterygoid canal and then through the sphenopalatine ganglion (without synapsing) to the respiratory epithelium of the head. Hypersympathetic activity to the respiratory epithelium produces epithelial hyperplasia. Epithelial hyperplasia is characterized by increased numbers of goblet cells in relation to ciliated cells and encourages the production of profuse, thick, sticky, tenacious, slow-moving mucosal discharge.

III. TREATMENT

Medical treatment at an early stage usually includes a decongestant to symptomatically reduce the air resistance through the nasal passages and make breathing easier. This treatment is subjectively effective by constricting blood vessels in the nasal mucosa; but in the long run, it actually encourages the detrimental sympathetic effects listed in the previous paragraph. Sidney Harris said, "A bad physician treats the symptoms, a good physician treats the disease, and a rare physician treats the patient." The osteopathic curriculum strives to produce the "good and rare physician." It is often necessary to treat the symptoms, for various reasons, but know what will be gained and what may be lost by doing so.

The principles of osteopathic manipulative treatment (OMT) in helping the body heal itself are outlined in Osteopathic Medicine:[2]

1. OMT stimulates blood supply

25

2. OMT increases venous and lymphatic drainage of the organ systems possibly affected
3. OMT relieves muscle spasm, reducing restriction on breathing
4. OMT reduces reflex disturbances that may be impairing

    a. Vasomotor regulation
    b. The function of secondarily involved organs
    c. Other defense responses

5. OMT improves circulation to and from the reticuloendothelial system, to aid its responses to an invading agent"

Simple rib raising manipulation to the upper six ribs reduces the sensitivity of facilitated segments in the thoracic area and results in diminished sympathetic outflow to the mucosa of the nose, sinuses and bronchial tubes. Treatment of related joint somatic dysfunction reduces facilitation at the cord level by removing its somatic influence. Treatment of cervical myofascial dysfunction opens fascial pathways for lymphatic drainage and simultaneously influences posterior Chapman's points (suboccipital area) through somatovisceral reflex action. Because of the fascial ties and the proximity of the cervical sympathetic ganglia to the vertebral joints, treatment of somatic

CERVICAL SYMPATHETIC CHAIN

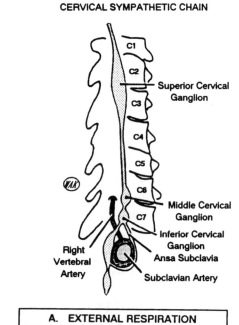

A. EXTERNAL RESPIRATION

ANTERIOR POINTS: DIAGNOSTIC AIDS:
UPPER RESPIRATORY TRACT (T1-4)

A. Ear
B. Nasal Sinuses
C. { Pharynx / Tonsils / Larynx }
D. Bronchus

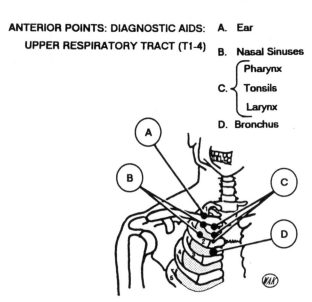

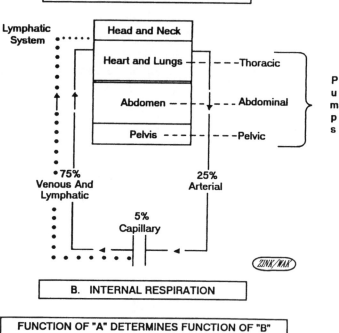

B. INTERNAL RESPIRATION

FUNCTION OF "A" DETERMINES FUNCTION OF "B"

26

dysfunction and fascial tension in the cervical area opens pathways for lymphatic drainage and reduces visceral afferent influences that are active in maintaining related facilitated cord segments. By reducing sympathetic influence and allowing the more desirable parasympathetic effects to predominate, the respiratory epithelium produces a thinner, more watery secretion. Treatment of this area first will also reduce the outflow of sympathetic impulses via facilitated upper cord segments.

Following treatment by rib raising, it is beneficial to turn the patient to his/her side and provide a kneading type soft tissue treatment to the thoracolumbar junction. This relaxes the patient and the lumbar attachments of the muscular abdominal diaphragm, preparing the patient for a diaphragm redoming treatment.

Increased interstitial fluid and mucosal swelling as a result of mucosal irritation, inflammation, and infection produces an exigency for effective lymphatic drainage to relieve congestion. Good lymphatic drainage requires unimpeded lymphatic pathways from the site of infection back to the heart and effective lymphatic pumping action from a well-domed abdominal diaphragm.

If not already accomplished, the following static landmarks should be examined at the thoracic inlet. Fascial torsion of the inlet should be diagnosed and effectively treated to remove any hindrance to this terminal drainage site for the left and right lymphatic ducts.

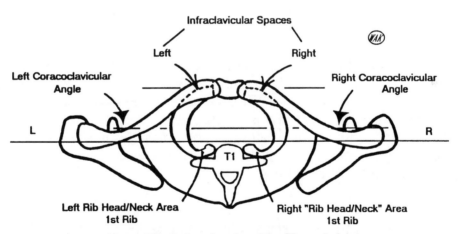

Normal Static Landmarks of the Thoracic Inlet

Diagnose and treat any somatic dysfunction in the midcervical and OA areas. This insures good phrenic nerve innervation to the diaphragm, relaxes the fascial pathways for lymph flow through the cervical area and can influence the parasympathetic response in respiration. The diaphragm is then redomed by any one of a number of indirect or direct fascial manipulative techniques. (See pages 212-217 in the treatment section of this book.)

With lymphatic pathways freed and the diaphragm redomed, lymph flow is initiated by using one of the many manipulative lymphatic pump procedures. The pectoralis lift treatment applied for 2 minutes furnishes the pumping effect of about 5 minutes of the usual intermittent chest pump treatment. This technique is also applicable to patients with osteoporosis, metastatic disease, various types of postsurgical conditions and also OB patients with tender, hypertrophied breasts. The pectoralis lift can often be safely taught to the patient's family for their use on the patient at home. In addition to moving fluids, the thoracic lymphatic pump has been shown to modify immune function.[3,4]

Attention is then directed to the face and sinus areas. The physician's fingers are placed over the infraorbital, and later the supraorbital, foramina. The skin and subcutaneous tissues are contacted and circular treatment is provided over the nerve branches of the trigeminal nerve as they emerge from the maxillary and frontal sinuses, respectively. These nerves provide the impulses which are interpreted as pain from the respiratory epithelium of the sinuses. When the sinuses are infected, the patient will be very sensitive to pressure over these nerves as they exit from their foramina, a helpful clue to the diagnosis of sinusitis. If these areas are not tender to the patient, "sinus treatment" is probably not indicated. Though the treatment is initially uncomfortable in patients with sinusitis, reasonable manipulative effort over these nerves helps to relieve the subject's "sinus pain." Effleurage to the face often completes lymphatic treatment.

Addition of a type of cranial treatment employs a frontonasal suture spread[5] and encourages the ethmoid bone of the skull to move freely and normally in the ethmoid notch of the frontal bone. Good functional motion of the ethmoid and frontal bones encourages a natural pumping action through the craniosacral mechanism and improves sinus drainage. This cranial technique may be incorporated by osteopathic students and physicians, even without having complete training in the craniosacral concept.

In order to influence parasympathetic outflow to the sinus and nasal respiratory epithelium it is efficacious to take a minute and treat the right and the left sphenopalatine ganglia. This treatment has two main effects:

o .. Parasympathetic activity is a primary influence in the production of a thinner, saliva-like secretion. Stimulation of this parasympathetic ganglion provides an "internal irrigation" by thinning the thickened nasal secretions and thus providing both symptomatic relief and improved regional homeostasis.

o .. It encourages the autonomic system to establish a more normal cellular ratio in the mucosal epithelium between the goblet and the ciliated columnar epithelial cells. Parasympathetic impulses reduce the goblet cells and increase the proportion of ciliated columnar cells.

The sphenopalatine ganglion is located in the sphenopalatine fossa of the skull and hangs from the maxillary division of the trigeminal nerve. This is a parasympathetic ganglion and it cannot be reached directly by the palpating finger. It may be reached indirectly, through the open mouth of the patient, by passing a cotted finger over the molars of the upper jaw, then lateral and posterior to the maxillary ridge and then cephalad over the pterygoid plates (just posterior to the maxillary ridge) to the extent permitted by the buccal mucosa in the mouth.[6] The patient is then asked to nod toward the palpating finger. Two or three repetitions on each side of the mouth provides adequate treatment by indirectly applying tension on the ganglion through the fascias of the pterygoid muscles. Satisfactory treatment is signaled by tearing of the eye only on the side of treatment, because the lacrimal gland shares the same parasympathetic nerve supply.

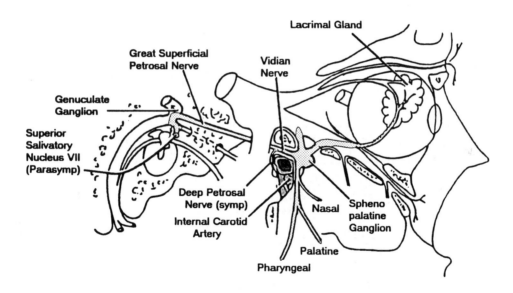

IV. SUMMARY

The osteopathic approach has been reported[7] to decrease the symptoms and duration of colds, to support the body's homeostatic mechanisms against infection, and to prevent complications and recurrence. Osteopathic manipulation provides increased comfort for the patient, balances and supports physiologic protective and homeostatic mechanisms of the body, and provides rewarding treatment for a patient with the common cold.

This section encourages the student of an osteopathic approach to understand, incorporate, and record the following:

o .. The sympathetic and parasympathetic innervation to structures of the head and the effects of each upon the respiratory epithelium and discharge of the upper respiratory tract
o .. The lymphatic drainage pattern from the upper respiratory tract
o .. Manipulative techniques for treatment of the thoracic inlet, redoming the diaphragm and initiating lymphatic flow
o .. Manipulative technique for applying effleurage of the face
o .. Sphenopalatine ganglion intraoral finger manipulative technique
o .. The diagnosis and osteopathic treatment of cervical, rib, thoracic, and thoracolumbar somatic dysfunction is indicated to remove the somatic component of the facilitated spinal cord segments including occipital (condylar) decompression, frontal/nasal spread, and CV4 techniques

---

REFERENCES:
1. Zirul EE: Infections caused by viruses, in Hoag JM Osteopathic Medicine. New York, McGraw-Hill, 1969, ch 45, p 722.
2. Op cit p 720.
3. Measel JW, Jr: The effect of the lymphatic pump on the immune response: I. Preliminary studies on the antibody response to pneumococcal polysaccharide assayed by bacterial agglutination and passive hemagglutination, JAOA Sept 1982; 82(1):59-62.
4. Measel JW, Kafity AA: The effect of the lymphatic pump on the band T cells in peripheral blood (abst). JAOA; 608.
5. Magoun HI: Osteopathy in the Cranial Field. Kirksville, Journal Printing Co, 3rd ed, 1976, pp 172, 290.
6. Op cit p 216.
7. Schmidt IC: Osteopathic manipulative therapy as a primary factor in the management of upper, middle, and pararespiratory infections. JAOA Feb 1982; 81: 382-8.

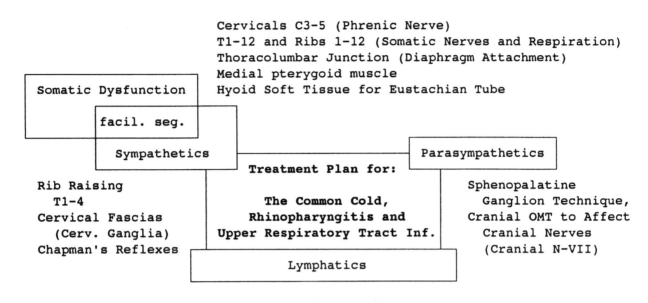

Cervicals C3-5 (Phrenic Nerve)
T1-12 and Ribs 1-12 (Somatic Nerves and Respiration)
Thoracolumbar Junction (Diaphragm Attachment)
Medial pterygoid muscle
Hyoid Soft Tissue for Eustachian Tube

Somatic Dysfunction

facil. seg.

Sympathetics

Parasympathetics

Treatment Plan for:

**The Common Cold,
Rhinopharyngitis and
Upper Respiratory Tract Inf.**

Rib Raising
  T1-4
Cervical Fascias
  (Cerv. Ganglia)
Chapman's Reflexes

Sphenopalatine
  Ganglion Technique,
Cranial OMT to Affect
  Cranial Nerves
  (Cranial N-VII)

Lymphatics

Thoracic Inlets
Abdominal Diaphragm
Effleurage
Lymphatic Pumps

SYMPATHETIC EFFECTS

↑ Tone:

    ↑ Vasoconstriction
    ↑ Thickens Secretions (↑ Number of Goblet Cells)
    ↓ Drainage

LYMPHATIC EFFECTS

Impaired Lymph Flow:

    ↓ Drainage
    ↑ Congestion

PARASYMPATHETIC EFFECTS

↑ Tone:

    ↑ Thinning of Secretions
    Improved Drainage

NOTES:

OSTEOPATHIC CONSIDERATIONS IN
THE LOWER RESPIRATORY DISORDERS

I. NORMAL FUNCTIONAL RESPIRATION:

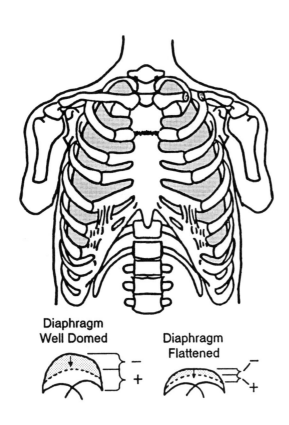

Diaphragm
Well Domed

Diaphragm
Flattened

Respiration is a dynamic orchestration involving coordinated reflex neural activity, abdominal diaphragmatic and various other muscular contractions, motion of fascial planes, and the movement of over 146 joints of the body. Efficiency of this orchestration is necessary for effective inhalation and exhalation, respiration and for the production of pressure gradients between the thoracic and abdominal cavities. The cyclic pressure gradients act as a pump for the lymphatic system and encourage good flow of lymphatic fluids. It is also involved in aiding venous flow and a host of biochemical and physical reactions occurring in the blood stream during respiration.

Breathing and respiration are not the same. The purpose of "breathing" is to move air from outside the body into the lungs, exchange oxygen in the air for carbon dioxide in the blood stream, and then exhale the air. The purpose of "respiration" is to provide for a similar exchange of these gases at the cellular level. If this is to be accomplished with optimal clinical effect, breathing must be coupled with good circulation in an interstitial tissue environment as free from congestion as possible. The lung maintains its internal environment and function via viscerovisceral and viscerosomatic reflexes.

Metabolic or respiratory acidosis or alkalosis results in a change of the blood's pH and affects its hemoglobin-oxygen dissociation curves. This means that the ability of hemoglobin to give up its oxygen to the cells will vary according to the blood's pCO^2 and serum pH. Even small increases in oxygen to the tissues is accompanied by a very great increase in protection of those tissues from infection.

Niinikoski stated: "Any treatment that augments the local oxygen supply or helps to avoid hypoperfusion tends to increase the rate of healing and decrease susceptibility to infection." Osteopathic manipulative treatment affects the pulmonary environment through somatosomatic and somatovisceral reflexes. It also affects the musculoskeletal mechanics involved in breathing, respiration and lymph flow. These mechanisms have been researched by such scientists as Burns, Hix, Olwen Gutensohn, Denslow, Korr, Krogh, Patterson, and Sato just to name a few.

Decongestion of interstitial tissues and improvement of respiration through mechanical and neuroreflex mechanisms are also encouraged by osteopathic manipulation.

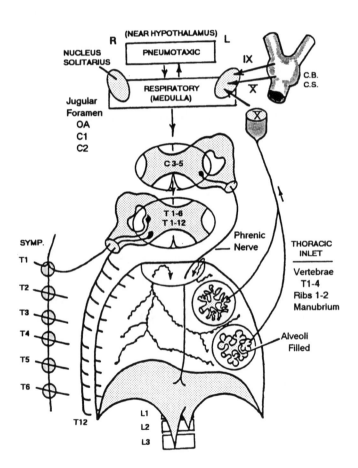

Through improvement of the body's fascial pathways and its own self-regulatory mechanisms for protection and homeostasis, electrolyte balance, pH adjustment, and the delivery of oxygen to the tissues occurs more easily and optimal tissue resistance and repair capabilities are encouraged.

In normal respiratory activity, the solitary nucleus of the respiratory center in the medulla is informed of the collapse of the air sacs by way of visceral afferent nerve fibers.

34

These visceral afferents travel in the pathways of the vagus nerve. The reflex response by the nucleus solitarius and the respiratory center in the medulla may be modified by impulses received from the carotid body. The carotid body is sensitive to CO_2 concentrations in the blood.

A subsequent reflex arch from the nucleus solitarius to the mid-cervical area, (C3,4,5) produces a contraction of the diaphragm via the phrenic nerve.

Somatic intercostal nerves, T1-12, are also called into action by this reflex producing stabilization of the intercostal spaces but doing little to move the ribs unless there is a call for very deep inhalation.

When the air sacs are filled, visceral afferent reflexes inhibit the nucleus solitarius and the somatic reflex pathways cause the diaphragm and intercostal muscles to relax.

o .. If the air sacs remain partially distended, the person's breathing may become more shallow.
o .. If the serum carbon dioxide content is increased, as in respiratory acidosis, viscerosomatic reflexes are initiated by the carotid body which result in an increase in the rate of respiration.
o .. The result of these two actions is a patient with shallow, rapid respirations.

The tubular bronchial system is lined with special pseudostratified columnar, ciliated epithelium which is supposed to protect and maintain the internal environment of those passageways. It is important to remember that it is the resultant balance between the sympathetic and parasympathetic nerve impulses to the lung that determines the cellular make-up of the respiratory epithelium. This means, especially, "the ratio of ciliated to goblet cells" in the lining of the bronchial tubes. It is this ratio which determines the basic type of bronchial secretions produced by the respiratory epithelium and thus determines the functional and protective environment at the mucosal bronchial membrane interface of respiration.

Parasympathetic influence via the vagus nerves is dominant in a normal functioning lung. The cellular ratio of the bronchial epithelium is dependent upon this parasympathetic dominance to produce a clear, saliva-like (but sticky) mucous blanket. This type of mucous blanket is easily moved cephalad toward the epiglottis by the action of the ciliated cells in the respiratory epithelium and it keeps the bronchial passages moist and clean. Because of the dominant parasympathetic:sympathetic influence in healthy lungs, there is normally a slight increase in smooth muscle tone of the bronchial tubes.

II. PATHOPHYSIOLOGY - "REFLEX ACTION DURING INFECTION:"

Pulmonary disease, whether infectious or not, may be looked upon as the result of the disruption or undesirable response of one or more of the protective mechanisms. Any disruption of the mucosal blanket or irritation of the epithelial lining of the bronchial tubes will obviously change the bronchial environment. Constant dysfunction of the lung's normal reflex mechanisms is associated with predictable pathophysiologic events.[1] Infection--viral or bacterial--is one of the most common irritants of the respiratory mechanism, although bronchial irritation produced by smoking is probably very common and, unfortunately, is often unnoticed until cell changes have occurred.

Viral or bacterial infections produces local irritation of the bronchial epithelium. An inflammatory response is set up which may spread into the parenchymal tissue of the lung. Alveolar surfactant is reduced, exudate forms, and eventually congestion and even edema of lung tissue ensues. Hours or days later there is sloughing of some of the injured mucosa.

At this point, the patient has "tissue congestion" and possibly even some edema which begins a compromise of the lung's cellular function in the process of respiration. The stage is set for the "signs and symptoms" of an acute viral or bacterial bronchial infection.

The respiratory mucosa of the trachea and bronchi is relatively insensitive to pain, but the movement of mucus and cellular debris over raw areas in the bronchial tubes activate a cough reflex. A cough can produce pressure changes of up to 300 mmHg in the lung and can produce air velocity up to 500 mph. While coughing is usually produced by a protective reflex, it may also be damaging and dangerous to some patients and is a significant etiologic cause of exhalation rib somatic dysfunction.

SYMPATHETIC RESPONSES:

Beginning with lung dysfunction and mucosal irritation, visceral afferent nerve endings in the area of tissue injury are stimulated. This results in a visceral afferent bombardment of the spinal cord from the T1-6 cord levels. When the lungs are irritated, the six upper thoracic cord segments have been found, experimentally, to have low reflex thresholds which discharge easily. This ease of discharge is associated with the finding of sympathetic hyperactivity in the related lung tissue. Viscerosomatic and somatovisceral reflexes occur in these lowered threshold segments resulting in activation by emotional, somatic, or visceral stimuli that are unrelated to the lung. This low threshold phenomenon is termed facilitation.

Viscerosomatic reflexes are the viscera's contribution responsible for initiating the facilitated cord segments in this example. Viscerosomatic reflexes will also segmentally interact with nuclei of somatic nerves in the spinal cord to initiate reflexes which provide the physician with palpable joint and musculoskeletal indications of lung dysfunction. These increased secondary somatic impulses produce palpable musculoskeletal indications of visceral disease in the T1-6 area (especially T3-4 and somewhat preferentially on the left). Afferent impulses from these somatic dysfunctions become the somatic contribution to the support and prolongation of the facilitated cord segments. When the lung parenchyma is involved, the inflammatory condition can produce direct irritation of the chest wall and intercostal nerve with accompanying musculoskeletal dysfunction adjacent to the lobe(s) involved. This produces pleuritic pain and is often accompanied by a pleural friction rub which can be auscultated.

Primary visceral afferent activity is also felt to be responsible for the formation of secondary myofascial tender points called Chapman's reflexes.

Cardiopulmonary System (T1-6)

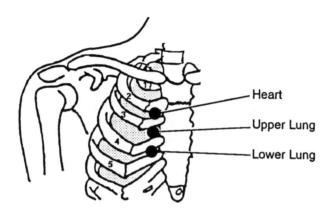

These points have distinct locations and can be used to help diagnose and then to adjunctively treat the visceral dysfunction of the lungs and other visceral organs. The anterior Chapman points for the upper lung and the lower lung are found in the third and fourth intercostal space, respectively, next to the sternum.

The sympathetic nervous system is involved in all disease processes. Prolonged sympathicotonia results in vasoconstriction with local hypoperfusion in the lung and epithelial hyperplasia. It even directly influences pulmonary immune function. Sodeman and Sodeman say: "The adaptive, protective reaction might be far more damaging to the individual than the noxious agent or the beginning dysfunction."

Hypersympathetic effects in the lung are initially responsible for some dilation of the bronchial tubes. This is not an undesirable effect at first; but persistence of the protective sympathetic responses is also responsible for a relative vasoconstriction of the arterioles in the area of tissue injury. Vasoconstriction along with interstitial tissue congestion encourages hypoperfusion of the lung tissues, the very tissues that need oxygen the most.

Another effect of hypersympathetic activity to the lung from the facilitated segment is a process called epithelial hyperplasia. In this situation, goblet cells in the bronchial epithelium increase. The ratio of goblet to ciliated cells increases. Not only is more mucus produced by the respiratory mucous blanket but the mucus becomes thick, profuse, tenacious and difficult to expectorate.

In this condition the patient not only has congested and edematous interstitial tissues, but also has thick, sticky, profuse tenacious mucus in the bronchial tubes. Edema of the distal air sacs may also be present in pneumonia, further decreasing the capacity of the respiratory system by partially filling the air sacs of the lung.

PARASYMPATHETIC RESPONSES:

It is known that the Hering-Breuer reflex mechanism cannot reflexly distinguish between air sacs filled with air and air sacs filled with fluid; so the respiratory center receives information from the vagus nerve to limit the excursion of the diaphragm because the air sacs are filled. At the same time the respiratory center receives information from the carotid body that more oxygen is needed and the abdominal diaphragmatic rate should be increased. The result is often shallow breathing at a rapid rate.

MUSCULOSKELETAL RESPONSE:

The mechanical and physical components of respiration are also stressed by the pathophysiologic changes just described. The diaphragm is mechanically stressed by relative immobility of ribs and spine (viscerosomatic reflexes) and also by the tissue resistance caused by congestion in the lung. Increased work load on the diaphragmatic muscle results in a strain of its attachments to the lower six ribs and the thoracolumbar junction producing an increase in the lumbar lordosis and a flattening of the dome of the diaphragm. The clinical result is often a patient with a spastic, flattened diaphragm that displaces very little volume during its contraction and relaxation.

Other palpatory clues to pulmonary dysfunction have been described.[2] T1-6 paraspinal tissues, and especially T3-4 on the left, have increased tone and are often tender from facilitation through viscerosomatic reflexes. T1-12 may have increased paraspinal tissue tone and tenderness when the lung parenchyma is involved. These musculoskeletal effects often restrict chest cage excursion and further diminish homeostasis. Another peak incidence of somatic dysfunction noted in numerous studies of patients with pulmonary disease can be palpated at C2.[3]

Coughing incorporates rapid contraction of the intercostal muscles. Persistent or unexpected coughing often results in exhalation somatic dysfunction of the ribs which then complicates the homeostatic response to the underlying pulmonary process involved. In severe chronic obstructive pulmonary disease, fatigue of the scalenes may result in depression of the first rib or exhalation somatic dysfunction of rib 2, otherwise infrequent findings.

LYMPHATIC SYSTEM RESPONSES:

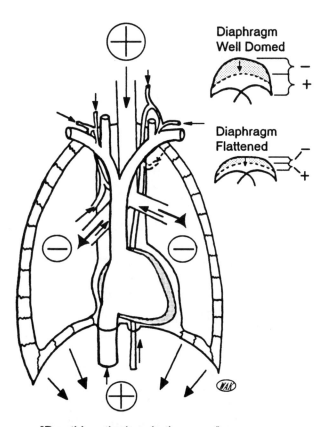

Diaphragm
Well Domed

Diaphragm
Flattened

"Breathing, the lymphatic pump."

Normally contractions of the abdominal diaphragm produce changes in volume between the thoracic and abdominal cavities. When the diaphragm is well domed, the volume changes produce effective pressure gradients between the thoracic and abdominal cavities. In this way a pump action for lymphatic flow is produced. Flattening of the diaphragm seriously decreases volume displacement and the pressure gradient that the diaphragm is able to produce between the thorax and abdominal cavities. In such a situation there is a decrease in the pressure between these two areas at any given moment. Decreased lymph flow increases congestion of tissues and can decrease cardiac output.

Under normal conditions, lymphatic return to the heart in a 24-hour period is equal to the entire serum volume of the body. There is no argument about the importance of maintaining lymphatic flow from the lungs in disease or in health.

39

Extrapleural lymphatics drain to intercostal vessels, to axillary nodes, and then into the left or right lymphatic duct; however, the drainage of the pleural sac and lung tissues travels to pretracheal nodes and then into the right lymphatic duct.

Basic medical and osteopathic research have proven that chronic lymphatic congestion with resultant poor oxygenation of the cells is associated with increased infection, increased mortality, increased healing time, and increased fibrosis and scarring if healing does occur. Studies have also shown that tissue congestion decreases the effectiveness of medical therapy. Respiratory therapy, pulmonary toilet and osteopathic manipulative treatment all have substantial effects on the prognosis of a patient when they are included in a program to enhance homeostasis.

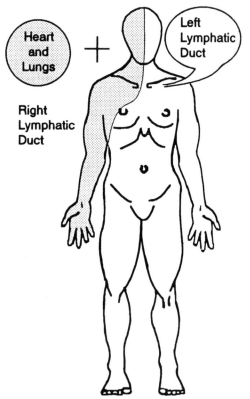

III. TREATMENT:

PNEUMONIA:

Lymphatic Drainage[4]

Lower respiratory infections such as pneumonia typically produce symptoms of high fever, hypoxia, tachypnea and toxic symptoms such as severe fatigue and headache; often the patient will initially have a repetitive, non-productive, non-effective cough. These patients may have chest pain, especially with deep inhalation.

It is also common to find patients with lower respiratory infections in which these typical symptoms are not present. This is especially common in the elderly patient. Their only complaints may be unexplained "toxic" fatigue, heaviness in the chest and/or a severe headache. Acceptable supportive care consists of bed rest to conserve energy, a light but nutritious diet with good fluid intake, and heat to the chest or the back. Fluid and electrolytes must be balanced and assured either by mouth or with intravenous drip.

Medical treatment consists of antibiotics, protection from non-productive cough, loosening of secretions, oxygen as required and occasionally bronchodilators. Early recognition of a lower respiratory tract infection is advantageous because this allows early institution of an antibiotic that is believed to be specific or of a broad enough spectrum before the cultures from deep expectorations and/or from the blood have been reported. When the cultures are returned, the result of the initial treatment is evaluated and the antibiotic changed if indicated. Palpatory and auscultatory physical findings precede radiographic changes by 24-48 hours.

Sometimes the cough may be suppressed by the use of dextromethorphan, codeine or other antitussive medications, especially if it is non-productive and damaging to the patient; sometimes antihistamines are given in hopes of making the patient more comfortable instead. Realize that these medications might make the secretions less fluid and more difficult to expectorate from the bronchial system. Treatment may be given to loosen the bronchial secretions and aid the patient's natural defenses. Mucolytic expectorants and proper hydration aid in the elimination of secretions and use of various mechanical means such as postural clopping and intermittent positive-pressure breathing procedures could be employed to reach this goal. Use of sympathomimetics to dilate bronchial passages allows the patient to breathe easier but the benefits of this type of medication must be weighed against the possibility of reducing blood flow to the parenchymal tissues of the lung.

The development of medications and antibiotic treatment for pneumonias has greatly reduced the patient's suffering from fever, hypoxia and systemic toxemia; and it has reduced the mortality from pneumonias. The effectiveness of these medications and the patient's comfort can be maximized by including an intelligent plan for osteopathic manipulative treatments in the patient's management program. These treatments need not be extensive to be effective; in fact, too much manipulation early in the toxic stages of the infection will tire the patient, reduce energy reserve and not enhance the treatment.[5] Suggested protocol and plans for providing osteopathic manipulative treatment to patients with pneumonia are presented on pages 45 and 50.

100,000 PEOPLE WITH VIRAL INFLUENZA IN THE 1918 EPIDEMIC		
	MEDICAL CARE	OSTEOPATHIC MANIPULATION
OVERALL MORTALITY	5%	0.25%
MORTALITY IF PNEUMONIA COMPLICATION	30-60%	10%

The effectiveness of osteopathic manipulative support for patients who were not receiving effective medications was clinically tested during the flu epidemic of 1918. Antibiotics had not yet been discovered to help patients fight bacterial complications. Even today, antibiotics are ineffective against viral infections.

In this study[6] of 100,000 people with influenza, Smith reported that patients who received osteopathic manipulation had a 0.25% overall mortality and a 10% mortality rate if they developed pneumonia. The mortality rates for patients who only received medical care and no osteopathic manipulation were 5% overall and 30-60% if they developed pneumonia.

Such a study would never be executed in today's scientific and effective medical society; but this early survey indicates the power and effectiveness of manipulative support of the body's own defenses. Combining medication with manipulative treatment to support body homeostasis has been shown effective in reducing the hospital stay length of stay by 10%.[7]

Initial manipulative treatment in pneumonia has three main goals: Reduce congestion, reduce sympathetic hyperactivity to the parenchyma of the lung, and reduce mechanical impediments to thoracic cage respiratory motions. Effective manipulative treatment accomplishing these three goals would also encourage removal of waste products for detoxification by the liver and removal by the kidneys; reduce vascular constriction in the tissue areas of the pathology; enhance more predictable antibiotic dose-to-tissue levels; improve respiration and make the patient more comfortable. These goals are addressed easily and efficiently applying basic manipulative treatment techniques.

Clinically, some variation of rib raising manipulation is commonly performed (see page 195) with special emphasis on the T1-6 area. The patient is usually supine and the head of the bed is elevated to provide ease in respiration for the comfort of the patient. Rib raising can be administered to one side at a time or both sides at once. The physician may also pass both hands under the patient's spine and grasp the erector spinae mass (ESM) with the fingers on one side of the ESM and the thenar and hypothenar eminences on the other side of the ESM. The physician's hands are then closed to produce tolerable inhibitory pressure on the erector spinae mass muscle. As this muscle group is grasped, the typical rib raising posture of the patient occurs with elevation of the sternum and ribs. While still grasping the muscle group; one hand or the other is adjusted by right or left displacement of the patient's spine until pressure between the two hands and the ESM of the patient seems to be as equal as possible. Hold this until the ESM muscles relax; then slowly release the pressures.

Rib raising not only relaxes the patient but is considered to effectively increase the blood supply to the lung tissues by inhibitory sympathetic interference with both vasomotor and bronchomotor control.[8] Prolonged hypersympathetic influence to the bronchial epithelium increases the ratio of goblet cells and encourages thick, sticky mucus. Effective rib raising should therefore reduce the results of excessively prolonged sympathetic influence on the respiratory mucosa, decrease the goblet cells in the mucosa and encourage a thin, saliva-like bronchial secretion. In addition to improving the arterial supply, rib raising enhances venous and lymphatic drainage from the bronchial and peribronchial tissues.[9] Rib raising techniques applied for about 30-90 seconds usually relax the paraspinal musculature and effectively treats sympathetic imbalance.

Manipulation is then directed toward improvement of lymphatic flow. The thoracic inlet is diagnosed for its fascial preference and is treated with indirect fascial manipulation or muscle energy direct techniques to produce freedom of fascial pathways in this terminal area of lymphatic drainage. Thoracic inlet somatic dysfunction can also be treated by thrust manipulation but the tissues of a toxic patient do not tolerate thrust activation as well. The thoracolumbar area is then relaxed with inhibition of the muscles in the erector spinae mass or by kneading the soft tissues, to prepare the musculature for redoming of the diaphragm. The abdominal diaphragm is then tested to determine whether both sides of this muscle are working effectively. The diaphragm is redomed if indicated using indirect or direct fascial methods with patient respiratory cooperation, breathing in or out and holding that phase of respiration as the physician directs the tissue release. A well-domed diaphragm produces greater pressure gradients between the chest and abdomen during contraction and relaxation; this indirectly results in greater efficiency in the movement of interstitial fluids by producing a more effective pumping action upon the fluids in the closed lymphatic system.

Mechanically the thoracic cage must be able to expand in all three planes for optimal breathing. Somatic dysfunction of any of the 146 joints involved in this process may be considered to limit maximal chest cage function and multiple sites of somatic dysfunction may provoke signs and symptoms.

The usual form of rhythmic compression and release of the rib cage to encourage movement of lymphatic fluids and even the pedal pump of Dalrymple may not be tolerated by an overly fatigued and toxic patient.

Lymphatic flow can be safely accomplished by grasping the pectoralis muscle near its tendinous attachment, pulling cephalad and slightly medially to tissue tolerance and then holding for a period of seconds or a minute or so. In effect, this procedure pulls superiorly on the attachments of the pectoralis major muscle to the upper seven ribs. With each inhalation by the patient this technique increases the volume of inhaled air. An additional 400 cc of air can be inhaled with each breath for each additional centimeter of chest cage diameter.

A=Ordinary Exhalation

B=Quiet Inhalation

C=Deep Inhalation

Exhalation rib somatic dysfunction particularly limits chest expansion, while causing pain and splinted breathing. Exhalation rib dysfunction is most frequently caused by coughing and therefore plays a major complicating role in many primary respiratory problems.

Lateral view of sternum with first and seventh ribs attached. The diagram illustrates motion of these structures during respiration.

Rib raising techniques may mobilize this dysfunction, but often specific OMT to the involved rib(s) is necessary to restore the homeostatic benefits obtained from effective breathing. Examination and treatment should not be limited to rib dysfunction however; OMT to restore normal motion to the thoracic vertebrae, sternum, and even the shoulder girdle have all been shown to improve the depth of breathing and to reduce the work associated with that breath. These may be the only treatments performed at the initial visit unless the patient also has somatic dysfunction at the base of the occiput and/or in the upper cervical region.

Headache is not uncommon in patients with respiratory dysfunction and is often an obvious clue to the frequently found somatic dysfunction in this region. The vagus has connections with the first and second cervical nerves and this may be the functional connection between the lung problem and the symptom of headache. Manipulation of any cervical somatic dysfunction, especially of the OA or AA should make the patient more comfortable and also normalize parasympathetic influence to the lungs through the vagus nerve.

Treatment for the hypersympathetic activity that is found in every disease process is often treated first. Hypersympathetic activity to an organ is enhanced by a facilitation of the cord segments related to the sympathetic innervation for the affected organ. The cord segments become facilitated by direct visceral afferent bombardment from excessive afferent impulses originating in the irritated lung tissues. Manipulation at any other area of the spine would send impulses past these cord segments of low threshold and very likely produce an outburst of sympathetic impulses to the lung from those segments. Therefore in many instances, it is physiologically desirable to calm down the sensitivity of the facilitated segments before manipulating other areas.

On subsequent manipulative treatments the continued function of these areas is easily determined and treated as necessary. Other areas and types of treatment can then be given as indicated by the patient's symptoms and by examination of the patient. Administering soft tissue treatment to the paraspinal areas while communicating with the patient not only provides information needed by the physician and the patient but also provides a tonic effect, improves comfort and provides palpatory information to visceral areas needing support and palpatory evidence of the vitality of the patient. Liver pump and splenic pump[10] manipulation, carefully applied, are believed to encourage detoxification and have been shown to increase circulation of WBCs, respectively. Manipulation also tends to prevent the complication of constipation commonly produced by inactivity and systemic toxicity.

Osteopathic manipulation in the treatment program of a patient with lower respiratory infection improves the patient's comfort and supports that patient's own self-healing and protective mechanisms. Osteopathic manipulation is provided for the patient's needs and by understanding the stresses that a patient should encounter with a certain disease; there is not a specific list of techniques used for a patient with a systemic disease. Osteopathic manipulation to support the patient works synergistically with the medical program directed toward the infectious agent and/or the disease.

Staging a patient according to the severity of symptoms has been shown to be useful when planning an osteopathic manipulative treatment program which will be beneficial for a patient with pneumonia. The following is a suggested osteopathic manipulative treatment protocol for hospitalized patients with pneumonia:[11]

SAMPLE OF TREATMENT PROTOCOL FOR PNEUMONIA:

Manipulative treatment in the hospitalized patient with pneumonia is suggested at least daily and ideally, three times a day. Charts and suggestions are only guides and it is the physician's examination of each patient that makes the final determination of the systems that should be supported and the areas that require manipulative treatment.

STAGE I: Moderate distress, febrile, non-productive cough, usually mildly to moderately dehydrated, exhibiting some degree of electrolyte imbalance.

A. Rib raising to point of tissue release in the paravertebral area on each side. Begin with the area of greatest involvement. In lobar pneumonia this would correspond with the ribs in direct contiguity with the lobar region of involvement. With bronchial pneumonia the entire rib cage region from T1 through 12 is often involved.

B.   Bilateral soft tissue myofascial release of the thoracic inlet fascias and similar treatment to the upper thoracic subscapular muscular and fascial tensions.

C.   Bilateral inhibition of paravertebral muscles in the occipitoatlantal area and down at least to C5.

D.   Bilateral occipital pressures towards cranial extension (CV4) if able to provide this treatment properly, is useful especially if temperatures are 101-103°

STAGE II: Diminished distress, lysis of fever, early productive cough, restoration of fluids and electrolyte balance.

A.   Bilateral soft tissue myofascial release of subscapular muscles and fascia, rib raising by inhibition of paravertebral muscles to point of tissue effect. Address treatment especially to tissues which are most significantly effected as determined by palpation.

B.   Bilateral soft tissue myofascial release treatment to anterior cervical fascias.

C.   Bilateral soft tissue myofascial release treatment of the intercostal muscles and fascias.

D.   Specific mobilization of C7 to T4.

E.   Gentle inhibition of the superior cervical segment. Extend this treatment down to C5.

STAGE III: Convalescent, afebrile, productive cough, restoration of fluid and electrolytes balance has been accomplished.

A.   Rib raising each thoracic paravertebral area until tissue effect is palpable.

B.   Lymphatic pump either by bilateral pedal pressure or thoracic pump.

C.   Specific mobilization of segmental vertebral somatic dysfunction as indicated.

PREVENTION OF POSTOPERATIVE PULMONARY COMPLICATIONS:

The two most common postoperative complications are ileus and pulmonary dysfunction. Upper gastrointestinal (GI) surgery is more likely to result in postoperative pulmonary complications than lower GI surgery, probably due to the proximity of the surgery to the diaphragm. Somatic dysfunction (C3-5: phrenic nerve) can compromise respiratory homeostasis. Henshaw[12] demonstrates the importance of treating this area pre-operatively to prevent respiratory complications following GI surgery.

INCIDENCE OF POST-OPERATIVE
PULMONARY COMPLICATIONS

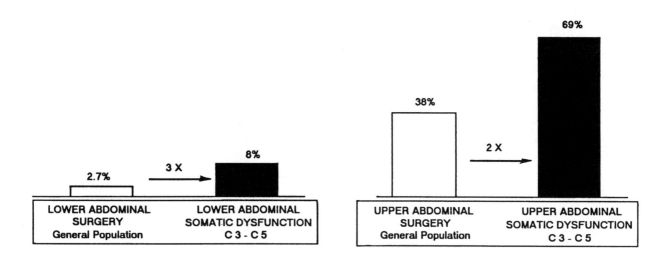

2.7%   3 X   8%

LOWER ABDOMINAL
SURGERY
General Population

LOWER ABDOMINAL
SOMATIC DYSFUNCTION
C 3 - C 5

38%   2 X   69%

UPPER ABDOMINAL
SURGERY
General Population

UPPER ABDOMINAL
SOMATIC DYSFUNCTION
C 3 - C 5

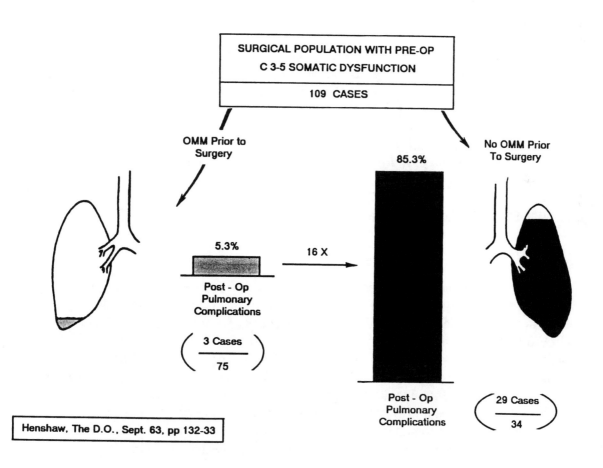

SURGICAL POPULATION WITH PRE-OP

C 3-5 SOMATIC DYSFUNCTION

109 CASES

OMM Prior to
Surgery

No OMM Prior
To Surgery

5.3%   16 X   85.3%

Post - Op
Pulmonary
Complications

$$\left(\frac{3 \text{ Cases}}{75} \right)$$

Post - Op
Pulmonary
Complications

$$\left(\frac{29 \text{ Cases}}{34} \right)$$

Henshaw, The D.O., Sept. 63, pp 132-33

CHRONIC OBSTRUCTIVE PULMONARY DISEASE (COPD):

Both functional and structural changes take place in chronic obstructive pulmonary disease that eventually affect the entire body unit. Hyperinflation with alveolar wall destruction leads to a reduction in the total alveolar area of the lungs and a concomitant loss of pulmonary capillaries. Hypoxia results and pulmonary vascular resistance is increased as is cardiac output. Pulmonary hypertension and right-sided heart failure may develop. Structurally, the patient usually develops a barrel chest and often the accessory muscles of respiration become over used. Hypertrophied scalenes may cause neurovascular compromise affecting the upper extremity.

The general guidelines discussed in the previous section on pneumonia are also applicable for supporting homeostasis in patients with chronic obstructive lung disease. Manipulative treatment to aid in chest cage motion, thoracic drainage, and diaphragmatic function are "extremely important"[13]. Somatic dysfunction in the upper thoracic and cervical areas is also treated to reduce segmental facilitation and to normalize autonomic activity important in both vasomotor and bronchomotor tone. With better blood flow to the involved tissues, COPD patients with properly managed somatic factors are clinically expected to require smaller and less frequent doses of medication.[14] Use of osteopathic manipulative treatment in COPD patients has been documented[15] to significantly benefit pCO_2, O_2 saturation, total lung capacity, and residual volume. In a study of chronic bronchitis patients,[16] 92% of the patients in the OMT group:

   - were able to walk greater distances
   - had fewer colds and upper respiratory tract infections
   - had less dyspnea

. . . than prior to their manipulative management.

ASTHMA:

Bronchial asthma is characterized by bronchospasm with trapping of both air and secretions leading to signs and symptoms of dyspnea, hypoxia, bronchial expiratory rales, and paroxysmal cough. The secretions are often excessively viscous and sputum is white, frothy, tenacious, mucoid, and shows microscopic eosinophils and Charcot-Leyden crystals. Both bronchospasm and increased bronchial secretions may be caused by overactivity of the bronchial branches of the vagus nerve.[17] Individuals that have hay fever or asthma therefore are generally vagotonic and also "are particularly prone to parasympathetic reflexes in the gastrointestinal tract."[18] Often patients with asthma also have high narrow palates corresponding to the extension cranial mechanics frequently associated with this respiratory problem.[19] Sudden stress factors -- emotional, physical, or environmental -- will often trigger an asthmatic attack.

In addition to identification of inciting factors with management aimed at avoidance or hyposensitization, various medications for prevention or symptomatic relief are utilized. In this section, however, only OMT will be discussed in detail. The "efficacy (of OMT) in asthma is particularly remarkable."[20] Stiles reports a 14% reduction in hospital length of stay (pre-DRG) when OMT was added to the medical management of asthmatic patients.[21] The text, Osteopathic Medicine, proposes the following:[22]

> "Rather than being merely adjunctive, osteopathic management of asthma is directed primarily toward the basic disturbance. Asthma is an outstanding example of a functional derangement. It dramatically illustrates how unbalanced homeostatic control can alter normal bronchial muscle tone, secretion, and vasomotor function to cause a seriously disabling state and ultimately, irreversible organic damage. The functional basis strongly suggests that somatovisceral reflexes may well be contributory or localizing causes. Such reflexes can convert subjective discomfort into a full-blown attack."

The goals for the use of osteopathic manipulative treatment during an attack may be dramatically different than the goals proposed for the use of OMT between attacks. During an attack, some clinicians may attempt to initially stimulate the sympathetics for the bronchodilator response that results and, carefully considering the significant spasm of the thoracic musculature induced by viscerosomatic reflexes, may assist breathing and respiration with a seated thoracic pump technique. The soft tissues should not be overtreated however. Pottenger notes[23] that either inhibition of the vagus or stimulation of the sympathetics are physiologically correct in addressing the patient with asthma. Other clinicians start with CV4 technique, correct the sphenobasilar extension mechanics, and manipulatate to normalize the vagus.[24]

Empirically, somatic dysfunction of the third or fourth rib is often demonstrated and, as with most viscerosomatic induced dysfunctions, responds poorly to high velocity, low amplitude techniques; other activating forces such as muscle energy or indirect methods can be quite effective. Treatment of the sphenopalatine ganglion may also be helpful.[25] OMT is believed to raise the threshold to irritating stimuli and to superimposed psychogenic disturbances.[26]

Between attacks, maximal thoracic, sternal, and costal motion is sought. Research by Perrin T. Wilson and by R.S. Koch demonstrated that OMT between acute asthmatic episodes is able to decrease the frequency and severity of attacks as well as the need for medications.[27]

BASIC PLAN FOR OSTEOPATHIC MANIPULATION OF PATIENTS WITH LOWER PULMONARY DYSFUNCTION:

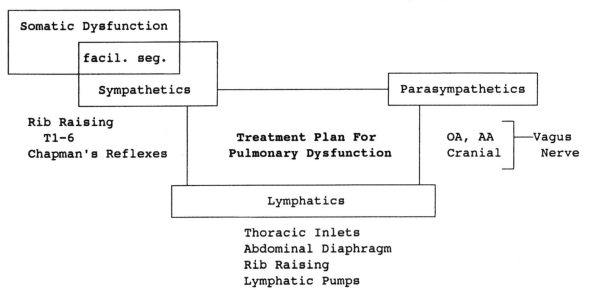

```
                              Cervicals C3-5 (Phrenic Nerve)
                              Sternum
                              T1-12 and Ribs 1-12 (Somatic Nerves and Respiration)
                              Thoracolumbar Junction (Diaphragm Attachment)

  ┌─────────────────────┐
  │ Somatic Dysfunction │
  │    ┌────────────────┴──────────┐                    ┌──────────────────┐
  └────┤   facil. seg.             │                    │ Parasympathetics │
       │   Sympathetics            ├────────────────────┤                  │
       └───────────────────────────┘                    └──────────────────┘
  Rib Raising                                              OA, AA      ─┐
    T1-6              Treatment Plan For                   Cranial      ├──Vagus
  Chapman's Reflexes  Pulmonary Dysfunction                            ─┘  Nerve
                 ┌────────────────────────────────┐
                 │          Lymphatics            │
                 └────────────────────────────────┘
                   Thoracic Inlets
                   Abdominal Diaphragm
                   Rib Raising
                   Lymphatic Pumps
```

SYMPATHETIC EFFECTS

↑ Tone:
   1. ↑ Thickening of Secretions
   2. ↑ Vasoconstriction to Lung Tissue
   3. ↑ Bronchiole Dilation

LYMPHATIC EFFECTS

Impaired Lymph Flow:
   1. ↑ Tissue Congestion

PARASYMPATHETIC EFFECTS

↑ Tone:
   1. Thinning of Secretions
   2. Profuse Secretions
   3. Relative Bronchiole constriction

IV. SUMMARY:

The ability to advantageously integrate and administer the combination of proper medical care and distinctive osteopathic manipulation to support the patient's respiratory system and compensatory mechanisms, depends upon a combination of these factors:

o .. the osteopathic physician's understanding of normal and altered reflex patterns
o .. the pathophysiologic properties of the disease
o .. the ability of the physician to evaluate the patient's individual reaction to the disease process
o .. the physician's knowledge and skills to provide effective and efficient manipulative techniques which will reduce hypersympathetic tone, remove biomechanical impediments to optimum chest cage motion, improve diaphragmatic function, move lymphatic fluids, and ensure more appropriate parasympathetic responses so that they can be provided for the patient when indicated.

A physician must treat the patient according to the present and future needs of that patient indicated by a physical examination, the estimation of impending stresses, the pathophysiological nature of the disease and according to that physician's training, belief, and knowledge regarding body homeostasis and the direct interrelationship of structure and function.

REFERENCES:

1. Killough, JH: Protective Mechanisms of the Lungs; Pulmonary Disease; Pleural Disease, in Sodeman and Sodeman's (ed) Pathologic Physiology. Philadelphia, W.B. Saunders Company, 1979, ch 16, p 455
2. Beal MC, Morlock JW: Somatic dysfunction associated with pulmonary disease. JAOA Oct 1984; 84(2): 179-183.
3. Ibid
4. Killough, JH: Protective Mechanisms of the Lungs; Pulmonary Disease; Pleural Disease, in Sodeman and Sodeman's (ed) Pathologic Physiology. Philadelphia, W.B. Saunders Company, 1979, ch 16, p 452
5. D'Alonzo AF, Evans DJ: Disorders of the respiratory system, in Hoag JM (ed) Osteopathic Medicine. New York, McGraw-Hill, 1969, ch 29, p 465.
6. Death statistics reveal comparative values of osteopath and drug treatments. Osteopathic Physician December 1918; 34: 1-2.
    and Osteopathy's epidemic record. Osteopathic Physician July 1919; 33: 1.
7. Fitzgerald M, (Stiles E): Osteopathic hospitals' solution to DRGs may be OMT. The DO Nov 1984: 97-101.

8. D'Alonzo AF, Evans DJ: Disorders of the respiratory system, in Hoag JM (ed) <u>Osteopathic Medicine</u>. New York, McGraw-Hill, 1969, ch 29, p 476.
9. Ibid
10. Purse FM: Infectious diseases in children, in Hoag JM (ed) <u>Osteopathic Medicine</u>. New York, McGraw-Hill, 1969, ch 49, pp 747, 751.
11. Chila, T: (Adapted from a clinical research project in pneumonia), OU-COM Department of General Practice.
12. Henshaw <u>The D.O</u>. Sept 1963; 132-133.
13. D'Alonzo AF, Evans DJ: Disorders of the respiratory system, in Hoag JM (ed) <u>Osteopathic Medicine</u>. New York, McGraw-Hill, 1969, ch 29, pp 464-465.
14. Stiles E: Manipulative management of chronic lung disease. <u>Osteopathic Annals</u> Aug 1981; 9(8): 300-304.
15. Howell RK, Allen TW, Kappler RE: The influence of osteopathic manipulative therapy in the management of patients with chronic obstructive lung disease. <u>JAOA</u> Apr 1975; 74: 757-760.
16. Magoun HW: Neuroscience studies, in Goldstein M (ed) <u>The Research Status of Spinal Manipulative Therapy</u>, Bethesda MD, US Department of Health, Education and Welfare (NINCDS Monograph #15), 1975, pp 295, 301.
17. Pottenger FM <u>Symptoms of Visceral Disease</u>. St Louis, CV Mosby Co, 7th ed, 1953, p 124.
18. Op cit p 270.
19. Magoun HI <u>Osteopathy in the Cranial Field</u>. Kirksville, Journal Printing Co, 3rd ed, 1976, p 268.
20. Umanzio CB: The allergic response, in Hoag JM <u>Osteopathic Medicine</u>. New York, McGraw-Hill, 1969, ch 43, p 693.
21. Fitzgerald M, (Stiles E): Osteopathic hospitals' solution to DRGs may be OMT. <u>The DO</u> Nov 1984: 97-101.
22. Umanzio CB: The allergic response, in Hoag JM (ed) <u>Osteopathic Medicine</u>. New York, McGraw-Hill, 1969, ch 43, p 696.
23. Pottenger FM <u>Symptoms of Visceral Disease</u>. St Louis, CV Mosby Co, 7th ed, 1953, p 125.
24. Magoun HI <u>Osteopathy in the Cranial Field</u>. Kirksville, Journal Printing Co, 3rd ed, 1976, p 268.
25. Op cit p 268.
26. Umanzio CB: The allergic response, in Hoag JM (ed) <u>Osteopathic Medicine</u>. New York, McGraw-Hill, 1969, ch 43, p 696.
27. Northup GW (ed) <u>Osteopathic Research: Growth and Development</u>. AOA, 1987, pp 82-83.

OSTEOPATHIC CONSIDERATIONS
IN CARDIOVASCULAR DISORDERS

I. INTRODUCTION

"The rule of the artery is supreme."
-- A. T. Still

The autonomic and lymphatic systems and their effects upon the function of the cardiovascular system have probably been studied more extensively than any other system. This is reflective of the significant impact that these elements have in cardiovascular function and the support of cardiovascular homeostasis in patients with severe compromise. Osteopathic manipulative treatment (OMT) has been shown by Stiles to significantly decrease both the mortality and the morbidity of patients with cardiovascular diseases and dysfunctions.[1] Rogers reports that OMT has been demonstrated to be of significant value in some patients with coronary insufficiency.[2]

This section briefly outlines considerations relevant in hypertension and atherosclerosis, cardiac arrhythmias, congestive heart failure, and myocardial infarction. Modalities such as diet, medication, exercise, stress reduction and cessation of smoking have great relevance to the complete osteopathic treatment program and these should be integrated into a total treatment program for the patient; however, in this chapter only the manipulative elements will be considered in depth.

II. PATHOPHYSIOLOGY

SYMPATHETICS:

The sympathetic innervation of the heart has its origins in cord segments T1-6 with synapses occurring between pre-and post-ganglionic fibers in the upper thoracic and/or cervical chain ganglia. While not totally ipsilateral, there are definite right- and left-sided distributions of sympathetic fibers to the heart.

The fibers originating on the right tend to pass to the right deep cardiac plexus to innervate the right heart and the sinoatrial (SA) node. Hypersympathetic activity to these right-sided fibers predisposes to supraventricular tachyarrhythmias.

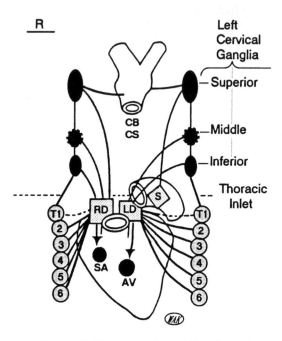

Sympathetic Innervation of the Heart

The fibers originating on the left tend to innervate the left deep cardiac plexus and the atrioventricular (AV) nodes. Hypersympathetic activity of these fibers predisposes to ectopic foci and ventricular fibrillation.[3] Sympathetic stimulation of selected fibers may increase the force of the heart beat, shorten the time of systole, increase ventricular output and increase the rate of contraction of the heart muscle without increasing blood pressure or raise the blood pressure without a general change in vasomotor tone of the body. Asymmetries in sympathetic tone may play a role in the genesis of serious arrhythmias.[4]

Increased sympathetic tone increases morbidity following myocardial infarction, it inhibits the development of collateral circulation, and it can adversely affect the degree of recovery from myocardial injury.[5] Increased sympathetic tone to the coronary vessels has been linked with coronary vasospasm.

Sympathetic nerve fibers are distributed to all blood vessels and generally cause constriction of the circular smooth muscles found in the vascular system. Sympathetic tone normally maintains the majority of blood vessels constricted to one-half their maximum diameter and therefore reduction of sympathetic tone produces a relative vasodilation. An overview of the sympathetic supply to vessels of various regions is seen in the adjacent diagram.

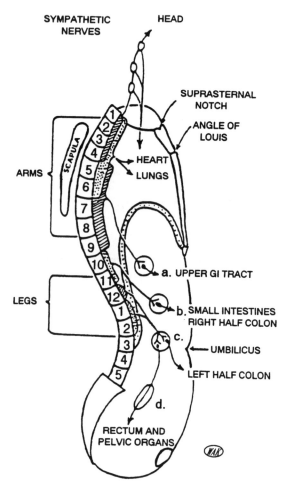

Sympathetic Innervation to Blood Vessels

54

Physiologically, these vasomotor nerves are generally unopposed and their activation typically produces vasoconstriction with reduced blood flow to the body tissues. Vasoconstriction can produce a shunt of blood from one area to another; and it usually increases total peripheral resistance and increases cardiac work-load. Veins are also constricted in response to sympathetic stimuli but the venous response is weaker than that in the arteries and arterioles. Sympathetic hyperactivity to the vascular supply of the kidney has been implicated as a possible cause of essential hypertension.

PARASYMPATHETICS:

Parasympathetic innervation to areas of the heart is also predominantly ipsilateral. The right vagus primarily innervates the heart through the sinoatrial (SA) node and its hyperactivity predisposes the heart to sinus bradyarrhythmias. The left vagus primarily innervates the heart through the atrioventricular (AV) node where hyperactivity predisposes to AV blocks. The heart may be reflexly slowed by stimulating the visceral afferents of selected organs. This seems to occur because of their common vagal innervation. Irritation of the pulmonary branches of the vagus produce the strongest inhibitory reflex influence on the heart. Irritation of the larynx, pressure on the carotid body or the pressure on the globe of the eye (oculocardiac reflex) will also reflexly slow the heart from stimulation of visceral afferents that activate vagal efferents. Normally, the oculocardiac reflex will provoke a slowing of 5-13 beats per minute; however, it will not slow the heart at all in sympathecotonic patients while slowing the heart 10-12 beats per minute in vagotonic patients.[6]

Somatic dysfunction of the occipitomastoid suture, OA, AA and/or C2 areas (where there are significant vagal connections) presumably produces effects through this afferent activation of vagal reflexes.

Parasympathetics are also involved in regulation of peripheral arteriolar vasculature, but only in a few select situations. In these areas the parasympathetic response in the local arterial vessels is vasodilation:

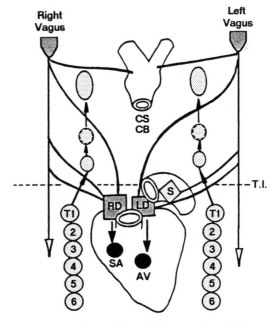

Parasympathetic (Vagal) Innervation of Heart

o .. submaxillary gland vessels via fibers in the small petrosal nerve (from
   cranial nerve VII)
o .. parotid gland vessels via fibers in the small petrosal nerve (from cranial
   nerve IX)
o .. vessels in the blush region of the face
o .. vessels in the tongue via the lingual nerve
o .. vessels of the penis via the nervus erigens

LYMPHATICS:

Lymphatic drainage from the heart and lungs is carried back to the heart
primarily by the right lymphatic duct.[7] Impaired lymphatic drainage from the
heart is known to severely compromise homeostasis and has been implicated in
reduced collateral circulation and increased morbidity and mortality from
ischemia and infection.[8]

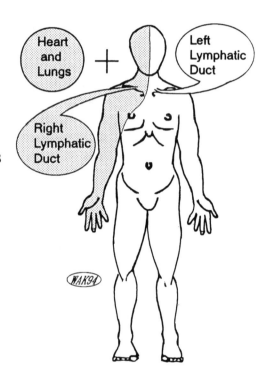

Congestion of cardiac tissues may result in
arrhythmias or changes in the EKG pattern
(sick sinus syndrome).[9] Peripherally
compromised lymphatic drainage has been
linked to the pathogenesis of atherosclerosis
and to the development of hypertension.[10]
It plays a significant role in pulmonary
edema, ascites, hepatomegaly, and the
peripheral edema seen in congestive heart
failure. Electrolyte imbalance which can
result from the development of peripheral
edema plays a significant role in the
morbidity seen in patients with congestive
heart failure.

The diameter of the thoracic duct and other large lymphatic channels is also
under sympathetic control. This fact should be considered in any treatment
protocol designed to improve lymphatic drainage. Hypersympathetic activity
can reduce lymphatic flow capacity.

SOMATIC SYSTEM:

Severe scoliosis with a thoracic curve greater than 75°, seriously compromises cardiac function. Other postural changes are more common and have their effects through somatovisceral reflex changes or segmental facilitation.

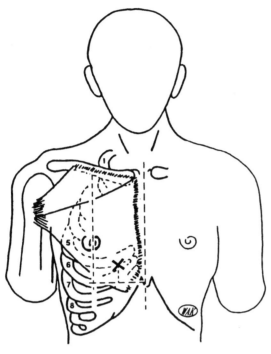

In our experience, patients with flattened thoracic kyphoses or with postural cross-overs in the upper thoracic spine tend to have periods of tachyarrhythmias when stressed. This is also the case in patients with a well-documented Travell triggerpoint located in the right pectoralis muscle.[11] This triggerpoint, in which posture may play an etiologic or perpetuating role, causes supraventricular tachyarrhythmias. When this is the etiology, the cardiac arrhythmia disappears when the triggerpoint is effectively treated.

Pectoralis "Arrhythmia" Trigger Point

Compensatory musculoskeletal problems may reflexly affect cardiac function. Treatment of the underlying postural stressor will usually be necessary before manipulative treatment of the compensatory somatic dysfunctions will result in lasting change.

Gait should also be analyzed and especially treated in patients with compromised functional activity from diminished cardiac output. Abnormal gait may increase cardiac work by up to 300%[12] and this may surpass the patient's energy reserves. Correction of an abnormal gait may allow a severely compromised patient to achieve a degree of independence in their activities of daily living.

Somatic factors also play a significant role in the differential diagnosis of perceived cardiac complaints. Anterior chest wall syndrome is often a generic term for any one of a variety of somatic elements which cause substernal and/or chest pains. Anterior chest wall syndrome is frequently misconstrued as

57

representing cardiac dysfunction. A partial list of specific entities falling into this category might include cervical, thoracic, sternal, or rib somatic dysfunction, costochondritis (Tietze's syndrome), intercostal neuritis, myofascial triggerpoints in pectoralis major, pectoralis minor, or sternalis muscles, or unrecognized rib fracture. It must be emphatically stated that somatic factors can co-exist with cardiac disease and that spinal segmental facilitation may augment the severity of one and/or the other. Correction of a diagnosed somatic problem, while it may relieve some of the cardiac symptomatology, cannot rule out the need for further cardiovascular diagnostics and/or therapeutics in a given patient.

REFERRED PATTERNS: can be referred from numerous sites

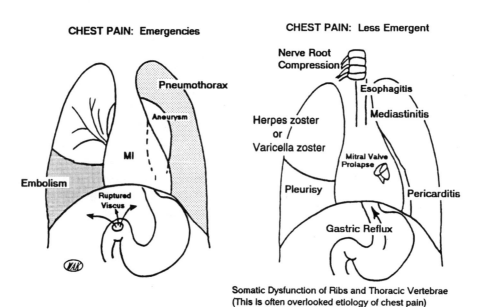

Somatic Dysfunction of Ribs and Thoracic Vertebrae
(This is often overlooked etiology of chest pain)

Pain patterns in somatic tissues from cardiac and coronary dysfunctions have also been well documented. Referred pain via the cardiac viscerosensory reflex from the coronary arteries (angina) is classically described as radiating to the upper half of the left chest, with referral out and down the inner surface of the arm and hand to the ends of the little and ring fingers. It may also refer up the neck and into the jaw.

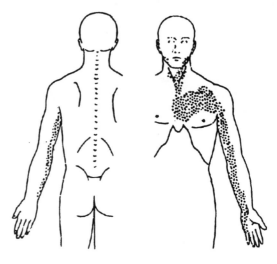

Referred Pain
Myocardial Infarction

This classic pain distribution into dermatomes C8-T3 is particularly true when the ventricle is involved; when the atria are involved, the pain is found lower in the chest wall, in areas of the T4-6 dermatomes.

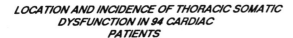

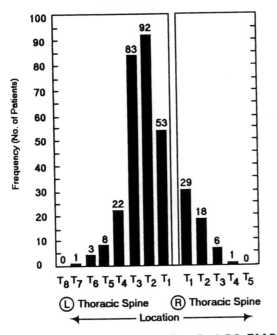

Adapted from data by Myron Beal, DO, FAAO "Palpatory Testing for Somatic Dysfunction in Patients with Cardiovascular Disease" JAOA 82 (11) pp. 822-831

Referral via the cardiac visceromotor reflex leads to muscular contraction and spasm in the upper intercostal muscles. Larson,[13] Beal,[14], and Nicholas,[15] as well as numerous other osteopathic physicians, have separately reported the consistency of palpatory changes primarily on the left side at the levels of T2,3,4 as being associated with cardiac disorders. Palpatory findings of somatic dysfunction at T1-5 on the left demonstrate 73%[16] to 79%[17] accuracy compared to angiography in determining the presence or absence of coronary artery disease. Chapman's reflexes from the heart are also consistent with these levels.[18] The posterior and inferior walls of the heart are heavily innervated by cholinergic fibers.

While anterior wall myocardial infarctions predictably demonstrate viscerosomatic changes in the T1-4 paraspinal musculoskeletal on the left,[19] posterior or inferior wall myocardial infarctions are accompanied by increased acetylcholine and bradyarrhythmias. Thoracic palpatory findings at T2 are less predictable in posterior and inferior wall infarctions. In myocardial infarction (especially with involvement of the posterior or inferior wall), these palpatory changes at C2[20] may need some explanation. According to some clinicians, an autonomic rationale can be postulated as an explanation because of the vagal connections to the C2 area.

The recurrent finding of somatic dysfunction or pain in the neck, cervicothoracic junction, upper thoracic area, chest, shoulder or arm should alert the physician to the possibility of a significant cardiac etiology. Likewise, while a myofascial triggerpoint in the pectoralis major may lead to functional cardiac changes, cardiac pathology may reflexly produce triggerpoints in the pectoralis myofascial tissues.[21]

III. TREATMENT SUMMARY -- SELECTED EXAMPLES

MYOCARDIAL INFARCTION:

The majority of patients seen within 30 minutes of acute myocardial infarction demonstrate signs of autonomic disturbance.[22] This is evidenced as sympathicotonia in the upper six thoracics (particularly T2-3 on the left) in patients with anterior infarction and as vagal hyperactivity (C2 and cranial base) in patients with inferior wall infarction. All MI patients would theoretically benefit from reducing the sympathetically associated cardiocardiac reflexes (C8-T5) so as to prevent ventricular arrhythmias; concern also exists for those with excessive parasympathetic activity which can lead to hypotension and subsequent diminished coronary blood flow to ischemic areas of the myocardium.[23]

For patients in the intensive care unit following myocardial infarction, patients with angina, or patients with other serious cardiac insults, treatment is therefore directed at calming the sympathetic hyperactivity especially in the upper thoracic spine to reduce inappropriate cardiocardiac reflexes, lower the incidence of ectopic foci and ventricular fibrillation, and to remove at least one factor which discourages development of collateral circulation. This is usually the first manipulative goal in the treatment sequence because ascending input from other manipulative techniques might otherwise be focused through facilitated segments into the injured myocardial region.

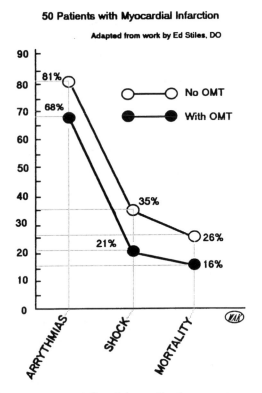

When integrated with effective medical management for this and other acute goals, specific osteopathic manipulative treatment should probably be limited to indirect techniques to avoid undue transient elevation of sympathetic activity to the heart from the treatment itself. OMT may also be applied in the form of generalized paraspinal inhibition to decrease total peripheral resistance[24] and cardiac workload.

Any thoracic inlet dysfunction is treated with indirect technique and if chest compressions have been applied during an emergency cardiac resuscitation, both the ribs and the sternum may benefit from indirect correction of the dysfunctions that are most certainly present. An excellent case can be made to also include treatment of hyoid dysfunction because of the fascial continuity to the mediastinum. Pectoral traction would probably be the treatment of choice to enhance lymphaticovenous return. The diaphragm may also be redomed using indirect techniques. Diagnosis and treatment of C2 superiorly including the base of the skull are performed in an attempt to address parasympathetic activity to the heart. CV4 is a technique that is helpful in fluid homeostasis as well as in lowering the patient's stress levels. Osteopathic manipulative treatment along the lines outlined in this section have been demonstrated to significantly lower the incidence of arrhythmias and mortality in post-MI patients[25] and to lower total peripheral resistance.[26]

Regardless of the techniques selected, a number of physiologic goals are considered to be addressed effectively by OMT. Thus OMT has been advocated for coronary heart disease by osteopathic manipulative specialists[27,28,29] and osteopathic cardiologists[30] alike.

ESSENTIAL HYPERTENSION:

Hypertension is a common problem affecting more than 15% of the US adult population. Of these cases, approximately 85% are considered to have primary or essential hypertension.

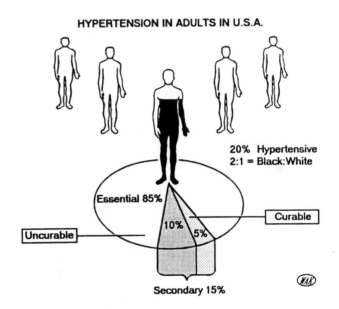

HYPERTENSION IN ADULTS IN U.S.A.

20% Hypertensive
2:1 = Black:White

Essential 85%

Curable

Uncurable

10% 5%

Secondary 15%

Most authors postulate essential hypertension to have a multifactorial etiology with a possible genetic predisposition aggravated by environmental and habitual factors as well as neurogenic, humoral, and vascular factors.

61

Functional elements are frequently implicated in the process:

o .. most patients with essential hypertension demonstrate vascular and cardiac hyper-reactivity to sympathetic stimuli;[31]

o .. prolonged sympathetic stimuli to the kidneys creates a functional retention of water and salt and elevated arterial pressure;

o .. venoconstriction is seen in the early labile phase of essential hypertension with an increased cardiac output accompanied by inappropriately normal peripheral resistance.[32]

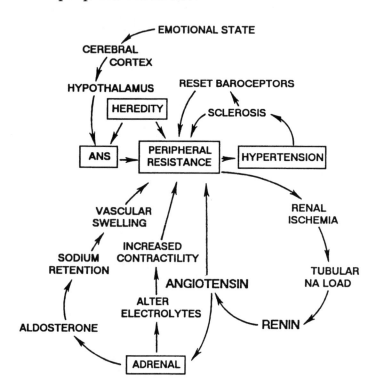

Eventually peripheral resistance increases and cardiac output returns to normal. With prolonged hypertension, the homeostatic mechanism incorporated in the carotid sinus baroreceptors resets and tends to maintain the increased arterial pressure.[33] The adjacent figure summarizes the physiologic factors involved in blood pressure regulation.

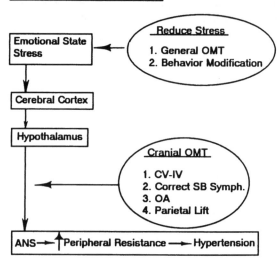

62

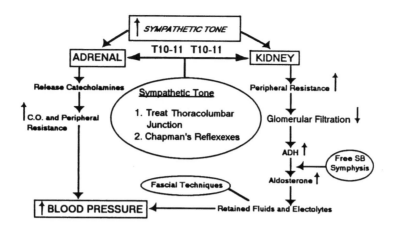

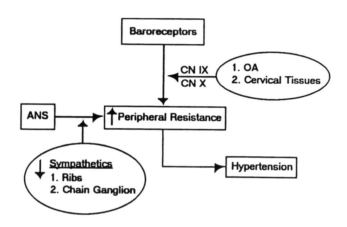

Based on physiologic mechanisms in these areas, OMT to support homeostasis should be effective in patients with hypertension. Regular osteopathic manipulative treatment is therefore felt to break the cycle of increasingly frequent episodes of sympathicotonia and delay the stage of fixed hypertension. According to Osteopathic Medicine, "Effective management of primary hypertension will postpone for years the time when compensatory mechanisms become exhausted and the effects of nephrosclerosis are manifested."[34] Due to the widespread distribution of the sympathetic nervous system, treatment is usually directed to the entire spinal column.

Stress reduction is extremely helpful in reducing cardiovascular manifestations especially in patients with evidence of the presence of facilitated spinal cord segments.

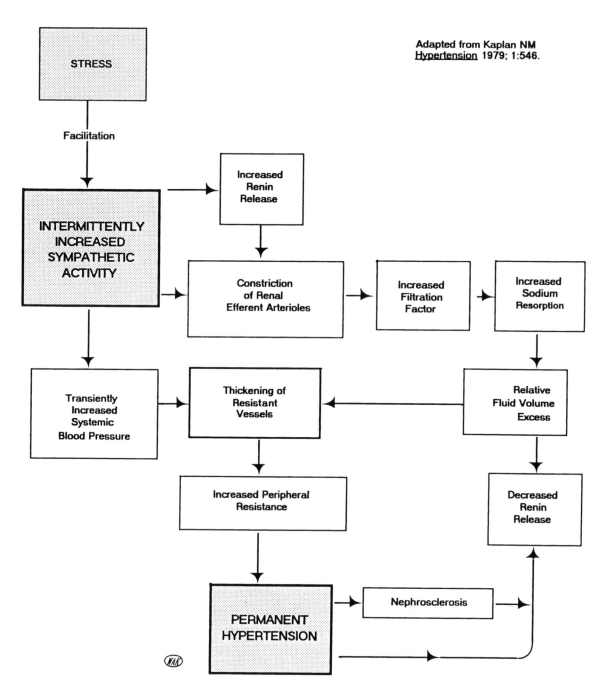

Adapted from Kaplan NM
Hypertension 1979; 1:546.

This diagram illustrates a hypothesis for the role of stress and the sympathetic nervous system in the pathogenesis of essential hypertension. It is adapted from Kaplan NM Hypertension 1979; 1:546.[35]

Patients with any cardiovascular dysfunction should also be given the benefit of treatment to address kidney and adrenal function because of these organs' intimate coordination in the maintenance of body homeostasis.

One study of hypertensive patients in which Chapman's posterior points to the adrenals were treated resulted in a blood pressure drop of 15 mm Hg systolic and 8 mm Hg diastolic pressure[36] and serum aldosterone levels in hypertensive patients have been demonstrated to decrease 36 hours post-OMT.[37] In another study of 100 hypertensive patients treated with OMT only, there was an average drop of 33 mm Hg systolic (from 199 to 166 mm Hg) and 9 mm Hg diastolic (from 123 to 114 mm Hg).[38]

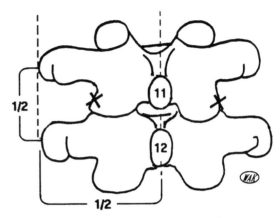

Rotatory stimulation of the posterior Chapman's points (T11-12) depicted above have been shown to effectively lower blood pressure and decrease serum aldosterone levels.[38]

Rotatory stimulation of the posterior adrenal Chapman's points depicted in the diagram above has been shown to effectively lower blood pressure and decrease serum aldosterone levels.[39]

Reduction of both systolic and diastolic blood pressure is the "rule" following OMT.[40] "Whatever technique is used, it should be slow-moving and gentle to augment rest and relaxation, promote autonomic balance and release fascial contractures."[41] The following chart postulates mechanisms for the treatment used in hypertensive patients based on the clinical results seen and the anatomic area being treated:

POSTULATED MECHANISMS FOR
OSTEOPATHIC MANIPULATION

TREATMENT	MECHANISMS	ONSET	FULL EFFECT
OA OCCIPITOMASTOID TECHNIQUE	NEURAL	30 SEC	30 SEC
RIBS GENERAL OMT BIOFEEDBACK	STRESS-RELAXATION; ANS	30 SEC	16 HRS.
THORACOLUMBAR JUNCTION CHAPMAN'S REFLEXES	RENIN-ANGIOTENSIN; ANS	2 MIN	?
FASCIAS CV4	BODY FLUID SHIFTS	10 MIN	1-2 DAYS

CONGESTIVE HEART FAILURE:

Physicians should place special emphasis on lymphatic goals when treating patients with congestive heart failure (CHF) in addition to the general approach to the autonomics discussed throughout this chapter. In CHF, 3 to 40 times the resting amount of lymphatic return challenges the system.[42,43] Dilation of the thoracic duct to several times its normal size may occur causing leakage out of the duct and subsequent ascites. Inability to accept further lymphatic fluid results in peripheral edema.

Increased venous and lymphatic return can be translated into increased cardiac output and homeostatic resistance to extension of injury following myocardial infarction. Optimal respiratory function is vital for the maintenance of treatment effects directed at lymphatic and venous return. For this reason additional time is felt to be well spent on treating diaphragmatic and thoracic cage somatic dysfunction. Lymphatic pumps and effleurage aid in fluid homeostasis and help to restore protein and electrolyte levels in these patients. OMT should not overload the circulatory system but may decrease the inefficiency of a dilated thoracic duct and restore lymphatic rates to resting physiologic levels purported to be maximal at approximately 1 ml per minute.

ARRHYTHMIAS:

> *"The comprehensive approach of osteopathic medicine seems peculiarly suited to cardiac arrhythmias. Chemotherapy can be lifesaving, but perhaps some of those life-threatening emergencies could be avoided if the physician would seek out and treat early sites of dysfunction however remote from the heart proper, or would view the onset of arrhythmia in the light of homeostatic and structural mechanisms.*"[44]

Rational osteopathic management including OMT is described in the text, <u>Osteopathic Medicine</u>, for sinus tachycardia, sinus bradycardia, sinoatrial block, atrioventricular block, extrasystole, paroxysmal atrial tachycardia, paroxysmal ventricular tachycardia, atrial flutter, atrial fibrillation, and conduction deficits.[45] Homeostatic support includes OMT directed towards reduction of segmental facilitation in the upper thoracics and use of techniques to modify vagal tonicity (such as pressure over the eyes, massaging the carotid sinus, strong forward bending of the head [Erben's reflex],[46] Valsalva maneuver, or treatment of occipital-OA-AA-C2 dysfunction). Structural support also includes appropriate attention to postural factors and correction of trigger points, especially those in the pectoralis (described on page 57) or sternalis muscles.

OSTEOPATHIC MANIPULATION OF A PATIENT WITH CARDIAC DYSFUNCTION

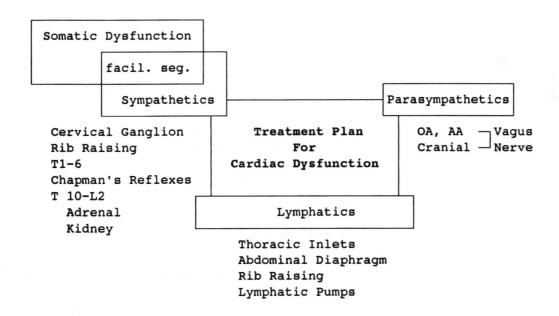

SYMPATHETIC EFFECTS

↑ Tone:

    1. ↑ Heart Rate and ↑ Vasoconstriction → ⎤ Increased
    2. ↑ Cardiac Irritability → Arrhythmias   ⎟ Cardiac
    3. Coronary Artery Vasospasm   ⎦ Work

↓ Tone:

    1. ↓ Venous Capacity
    2. ↓ Ability to Develop Collateral Circulation

LYMPHATIC EFFECTS

Impaired Flow:

    1. ↑ Central Venous Pressure
    2. ↑ Tissue Congestion → Decreased O_2 and Nutrients
       to the Myocardium
    3. ↑ In Size of Infarction from MI
    4. ↑ Risk of Subacute Bacterial Endocarditis

PARASYMPATHETIC EFFECTS

↑ Tone:

    1. Bradyarrhythmias via SA Node (Right Vagus)
    2. Heart Block via the AV Node (Left Vagus)
    3. Hypotension and Diminished Coronary Blood Flow
       in Inferior MI

IV. CLINICALLY RELEVANT ABSTRACTS - BIBLIOGRAPHY

The following section briefly abstracts a few points supportive of the postulated role that structure-function interrelationships and/or homeostatic factors play in an osteopathic approach to treatment of the cardiovascular system. The reader is encouraged to review the complete article for specifics or qualifications and to integrate their findings into the brief descriptions of osteopathic care offered in this chapter.

AUTONOMIC NERVOUS SYSTEM:

1. "The observation that in the majority of patients seen within 30 minutes after the onset of acute myocardial infarction there were signs of 'autonomic disturbance,' namely signs of sympathetic hyperactivity mostly in patients with anterior infarction and signs of vagal hyperactivity mostly in patients with inferior infarction, not only represented a major contribution but also provided a necessary link between experimental studies and clinical reality."[47]

2. Active visceral afferent impulses from the heart produce reflex effects which are mediated at spinal levels through a cardio-cardiac reflex (viscerovisceral) and are involved in extending the degree of myocardial injury in myocardial infarction. Occlusion of the left circumflex coronary artery in dogs lead to tachycardia. It was also observed that if denervation of the sympathetics was performed first and then a coronary artery was occluded, those dogs had smaller areas of myocardial infarction than dogs that were not denervated.[48]

3. "There is a link between the magnitude of sympathetic activity in humans with myocardial infarction and the heart muscle metabolism, and accompanying hemodynamics and clinical disorders. The nature of the adrenergic response remains mysterious. In particular, it is not known why this response (sympathicotonia) is large in one individual and only moderate in another."[49]

4. Stimulation of sympathetic nerves lowers the cardiac muscle's threshold for ventricular fibrillation in animals and has been seen to increase coronary vascular resistance in patients with ischemic heart disease.[50]

5. Sudden death is the result of ventricular fibrillation. This condition can be reversed if realized and if equipment is available for treatment. Transient risk factors induce electrical instability and in the electrically unstable heart there is increased susceptibility to ventricular fibrillation. These transient risk factors are generally derived from activities higher up in the nervous system:

o .. sympathetic pathways from the hypothalamus are implicated in the genesis of ventricular arrhythmias
o .. the left stellate ganglion is dominant in the enhancement of sympathetic efferent activity which predisposes to ventricular fibrillation
o .. stimulation of the left stellate ganglion is associated with increases in the inotropic effect to the heart while right-sided stellate stimulation increases both chronotropic and inotropic effects
o .. influence of circulating adrenal catecholamines on cardiac excitability is considerably less than the influence of the neural input to the heart from the stellate ganglion

In summary, increased sympathetic activity predisposes the heart to ventricular fibrillation. Protection can be achieved with surgical denervation, pharmacologic denervation, or procedures which reflexly reduce sympathetic tone.[51]

6. The most striking and convincing evidence that sympathetic neural inputs are active in provoking malignant ventricular arrhythmias is demonstrated by the series of disorders of ventricular repolarization known collectively as the long Q-T syndrome. A variety of sensory inputs, ranging from emotionally stressful

events to noise and exertion, may trigger ventricular tachycardia or ventricular fibrillation. An imbalance between the right and left stellate ganglionic sympathetic impulses to the heart has been postulated as being the mechanism responsible for this.[52]

7. A cardio-cardiac reflex takes place within a few seconds of ischemia and plays an important role in the genesis of early ventricular arrhythmias. Interruption of visceral afferents from C8-T5 reduces the arrhythmias to a major extent.[53]

8. On initial examination, patients with sinus tachycardia were found to have sympathetic overactivity.

Transient hypertension in the absence of sinus tachycardia was also regarded as evidence of sympathetic activity. Patients with sinus bradycardia or AV block were considered to have parasympathetic overactivity. Sympathetic and parasympathetic overactivity may coexist in cardiac patient.

The anatomical distribution of vagal receptors may explain the greater frequency of parasympathetic overactivity in patients with posterior infarction . . . reflex vagal overactivity may produce AV block.[54]

9. Experiments revealed that when sympathetic nerves to the kidneys are stimulated continuously for several weeks, fluid retention from reduced renal function occurs and results in chronically elevated arterial pressure as long as the sympathetic stimulation continues. It is therefore logically theorized that sympathetic stimulation of the kidney produces chronic elevation of arterial pressure.

Essential hypertension is probably produced by functional retention of water and salt by the kidneys.[55]

LYMPHATICS:

1. Respiratory activity is the principal mechanism underlying the flow of lymph from the thoracic duct into the venous system. It appears that the capacity for transfer of lymph is delicately adjusted to the normal rate of lymph production. Patients with systemic or portal venous circulatory congestion convert the plasma into lymph at an abnormally high rate. Available evidence indicates that this excessive volume of lymph, amounting at times to 3-4 times the blood volume in a 24 hour period, eventually exceeds the flow capacity of the thoracic duct/venous junction. The flow capacity of this junction appears to underlay distension of the duct and the formation of ascites."[56]

2. "Kellner in 1955 reported an interesting study of the relationship of lymph and its possible role in the pathogenesis of atherosclerosis."

"It seems likely that under normal circumstances there is a constant flow of fluid containing various serum lipids and protein across the endothelium into the walls of the blood vessels; this material normally passes through the wall and is completely removed by way of vasovasorum and lymphatics. In certain conditions, however, where there are increased amounts of lipid in the blood or where there are excessive quantities of certain types of lipids, the removal of these particles from the wall of the vessel is incomplete and some remain to initiate the process of atherosclerosis."

"In hypertension, increased hydrostatic pressure appears to cause an increase in the quantity of serolipoprotein that diffuses across the vessel wall, thereby increasing the possibility for incomplete removal and hence for the deposition of lipids."

"In this theoretical formulation of the pathogenesis of atherosclerosis, the artery wall is regarded as an organ which is constantly bathed by a serum transudate containing, among other things, various serolipoproteins, most of which pass on through, some of which doubtless are metabolized locally and a few of which remain behind to cause mischief."[57]

3. If by anatomic fault or abnormal physiologic mechanisms, lymphaticovenous communications fail to function, the rate of edema of the limbs or organs in congestive heart failure may be increased or resolution (including response to therapy) may be impeded.

"Data so far suggests that lymphaticovenous communications or, more broadly, adequate lymph flow plays a part in minimizing pathologic manifestations of disordered lymph flow from a particular organ or limb."[58]

4. There exists at present a "state of insufficient training of most physicians in lymphology."[59]

5. In a study[60] of 28 dogs and 10 humans: "Insufficiency of the cardiac lymph circulation has not only a theoretical but also clinical importance in the pathogenesis of arrhythmias."

In cardiac lymphostasis the following was observed:

o .. dilated lymph vessels, interstitial edema, edematous swelling of the myofibrils and changes in atrial action potentials
o .. shortened effective refractory period of atrium and ventricle (irritability)
o .. diminished SA node automatism

o .. slowed AV conduction (prolonged P-Q --> AV blocks)
o .. EKG changes similar to sick sinus syndrome

6. The protective role of the pulmonary lymphatic system is dramatically evident when there is an abrupt development of pulmonary edema in a previously asymptomatic patient with advanced mitral stenosis. These people develop congestive heart failure and often demonstrate a functional expansion of the pulmonary lymphatics over a period of time. The expansion with increased lymph flow may be a compensatory mechanism to remove the overt pulmonary edema.[61]

7. Experimental evidence by a team of cardiologists at Michael Reese Hospital (Chicago) notes: Fibrous and elastic tissue increases significantly in the ventricular endocardium when a dog's cardiac lymph flow is chronically impaired. Impairment of cardiac lymph flow may similarly cause endomyocardial fibrosis and endocardial fibroelastosis in humans.

Ventricular subendocardial hemorrhages frequently occurred soon after lymph flow obstruction in the heart of dogs. Areas of hemorrhage might lead to fibrosis when cardiac lymph drainage was chronically inadequate. Autologous blood injected into the left ventricle of lymph-impeded animals led to marked fibrosis and changes resembling the pathology seen after acute myocardial infarction. This was compared to few abnormalities found in controls with normal cardiac lymph flow.

Dogs with impaired cardiac lymph drainage were injected with bacteria and most developed endocarditis of the mitral valve. This was compared to no occurrences in controls with normal lymph flow. Researchers were lead to conclude that chronic interference with lymph flow predisposes to infection and inflammation. If impaired drainage from the heart is one of the factors that predispose a human to bacterial endocarditis, then "it is conceivable that this is one of the means by which rheumatic fever predisposes to subsequent bacterial infection."

It is unquestionable, the lymphatic system was important in the reparative processes seen in dogs after the injection of autologous blood into the myocardium and lymph flow may prove to be equally significant in healing after acute myocardial infarction. Animals with intact lymphatic drainage of the heart undergoing the same injection showed much smaller or absent areas of infarction and had a lower mortality and morbidity than animals with impaired lymphatic drainage.

Dr. Dumont of NY University studied the effect of cannulizing and venting nine patients who were in the final stages of heart disease and had huge distended thoracic ducts from lymph under pressure. Within 24 hours, central venous pressures fell toward normal and distended neck veins, peripheral edema, ascites and liver tenderness all diminished or disappeared. Liver edges no longer projected out under the costal margin.[62]

REFERENCES:

1. Fitzgerald M, (Stiles, E): Osteopathic hospitals' solution to DRGs may be OMT. The DO Nov 1984: 97-101.
2. Rogers JT, Rogers JC: The role of osteopathic manipulative therapy in the treatment of coronary heart disease. JAOA Sept 1976; 76: 71-81.
3. Corr PB, Gillis RA: Autonomic neural influences on the dysrhythmias resulting from myocardial infarction. Circ Research July 1978; 43(1): 1-9.
   and Lown B, Verrier RL, Rabinowitz SH: Neural and psychologic mechanisms and the problem of sudden cardiac death. Am J Cardio May 26, 1977; 39: 890-902.
4. Ibid (Lown et al.)
5. J Autonomic Nervous System, 1981.
6. Pottenger FM Symptoms of Visceral Disease. St Louis, CV Mosby Co, 7th ed, 1953, p 111.
7. Sodeman WA, Sodeman TM Pathologic Physiology: Mechanisms of Disease. Philadelphia, WB Saunders, Sixth Edition, 1979.
8. Miller AJ: The lymphatic system and cardiac disease, in Mayerson HS (ed) Lymph and the Lymphatic System, CC Thomas 1968, pp 213-229.
   and Lymphatics' role stressed in cardiovascular disease. Med World News Jan 21, 1966; pp 100-101.
9. Foldi Progress in Lymphology, pp 84-85.
10. Mayerson HS: One aspect of the role of the lymphatic system in cardiovascular function, in National Conference on Cardiovascular Diseases The Heart and Circulation. Washington, 1965, Vol 1, pp 90-91.
11. Travell JG, Simons DG Myofascial Pain and Dysfunction: A Trigger Point Manual. Baltimore, Williams & Wilkins, 1983, ch 42.
12. Saunders JB: The major determinants in normal and pathological gait. The Journal of Bone and Joint Surgery Jul 1953; 35-A(3): 543-558.
13. Larson NJ: Summary of site and occurence of paraspinal soft tissue changes of patients in the intensive care unit. JAOA May 1976; 75: 840-842.
14. Beal MC: Viscerosomatic reflexes: A review. JAOA Dec 1985: 786-801.
15. Nicholas AS, DeBias DA, Ehrenfeuchter W, England KM, England RW, Greene CH, Heilig D, Kirschbaum: A somatic component to myocardial infarction. Brit Med J July 6, 1985; 291: 13-17.
16. Cox JM, Gorbis S, Dick LM: Palpable musculoskeletal findings in coronary artery disease: Results of a double-blind study. JAOA Jul 1983; 82(11): 832-36.
17. Beal MC, Kleiber GE: Somatic dysfunction as a predictor of coronary artery disease. JAOA May 85; 85(5): 302-307.

18. Byrnes TR, Kuchera ML, Guffey JM, Steele KM, Beatty DR, Haman JL, Lockwood MD: Correlation of palpatory findings with visceral diagnoses. JAOA 92(9):1177, Sept 1992.
19. Rosero H et al: Correlation of palpatory observations with anatomic locus of acute myocardial infarction. JAOA Feb 1987; 87: 119.
20. Beal MC: Palpatory testing for somatic dysfunction in patients with cardiovascular disease. JAOA Jul 1983; 82(11): 822-831.
21. Travell JG, Simons DG Myofascial Pain and Dysfunction: The Trigger Point Manual, Williams & Wilkins, 1983, pp 585-586.
22. Schwartz PJ, Stone HL: The role of the autonomic nervous system in sudden coronary death. Annals NY Academy of Sciences 1982; 382:162-180.
23. Ibid
24. Burchett G, Dickey J, Kuchera M: Somatovisceral effects of osteopathic manipulative treatment on cardiovascular function in patients (abst). JAOA 1984; 84(1): 74.
25. Fitzgerald M, (Stiles E): Osteopathic hospitals' solution to DRGs may be OMT. The DO Nov 1984: 97-101.
26. Burchett G, Dickey J, and Kuchera M: Somatovisceral effects of osteopathic manipulative treatment on cardiovascular function in patients (abst). JAOA 1984; 84(1): 74.
27. Patriquin DA: Manipulation for the patient with myocardial infarction. Osteopathic Symposium February, 1975; pp 16-17.
28. Stookey JR: OMT for angina. Osteopathic Symposium March 1975; pp 16-18.
29. Frymann V: Osteopathic manipulation held to aid heart function. Clinical Trends in Osteopathic Medicine March-April 1976; pp 1, 5.
30. Rogers JT, Rogers JC: The role of osteopathic manipulative therapy in the treatment of coronary heart disease. JAOA Sept 1976, 76:71-81.
31. Merck Manual, Rahway NJ, MSD Research Lab, 15th ed, 1987, p 390.
32. Op cit p 393.
33. Op cit p 390.
34. Daiber WF: Disorders of the kidneys in Hoag JM (ed) Osteopathic Medicine. New York, McGraw-Hill, 1969, ch 39, pp 644-5.
35. Kaplan NM: Arterial hypertension, in Stein JH (ed) Internal Medicine. Boston, Little, Brown and Co, 3rd ed, 1990, p 240.
36. Mannino JR: The application of neurologic reflexes to the treatment of hypertension. JAOA; 79(10): 607-608.
37. Mannino JR: The application of neurologic reflexes to the treatment of hypertension. JAOA Dec 1979; 79: 225-231.
38. Northup TL: Manipulative management of hypertension. JAOA Aug 1961; 60: 973-978.
39. Mannino JR: The application of neurologic reflexes to the treatment of hypertension. JAOA Dec 1979; 79: 225-231.
40. Daiber WF: Disorders of the kidneys in Hoag JM (ed) Osteopathic Medicine. New York, McGraw-Hill, 1969, ch 39, p 655.
41. Magoun HI Osteopathy in the Cranial Field. Kirksville, Journal Printing Co, 3rd ed, 1976, p 280.

42. Dumont AE, Clauss RH, Reed GI: Lymph drainage in patients with congestive heart failure, comparison with findings in hepatic cirrhosis. NEJM 1963; 269:949-952.
43. Lymphatics' role stressed in cardiovascular disease. Med World News January 21, 1966: 100-101.
44. Baldwin W, Jr: Cardiac arrhythmias, in Hoag JM (ed) Osteopathic Medicine. New York, McGraw-Hill, 1969, ch 30, p 477.
45. Op cit pp 480-486.
46. Pottenger FM Symptoms of Visceral Disease. St Louis, CV Mosby Co, 7th ed, 1953, p 111.
47. Schwartz PJ, Stone HL: The role of the autonomic nervous system in sudden coronary death. Annals NY Acad Sci 1982; 82: 162-180.
48. J Autonomic Nervous System, 1981.
49. Circ Research 1981; 48: 6.
50. NEJM August 21, 1980.
51. Lown B, Verrier RL, Rabinowitz SH: Neural and psychologic mechanisms and the problem of sudden cardiac death. Am J Cardio 1977; 39: 890-902.
52. DeSilva RA: Central nervous system risk factors for sudden cardiac death. Annals NY Acad Sci 1982; 382: 143-161.
53. Schwartz PJ, Stone HL: The role of the autonomic nervous system in sudden coronary death. Annals NY Acad Sci 1982; 382: 162-180.
54. Autonomic disturbance at the onset of acute myocardial infarction. Neural Mechanisms in Cardiac Arrhythmias, 1978.
55. Guyton Textbook of Physiology.
56. Am J of the Med Sci 1975; 269: 3.
57. Mayerson HS: One aspect of the role of the lymphatic system in cardiovascular function, in National Conference on Cardiovascular Diseases The Heart and Circulation. Washington, 1965, vol 1, pp 90-91.
58. Threefoot S: Lymphaticovenous communications, in Lymph and the Lymphatic System. CC Thomas, 1968, ch 2.
59. Foldi Progress in Lymphology.
60. Op cit pp 84-85.
61. Mayerson HS Proceedings of the Conference on Lymph and the Lymphatic System. CC Thomas, 1968.
62. Miller AJ: The lymphatic system and cardiac disease, in Lymph and the Lymphatic System, CC Thomas, 1968, pp 217-229.
    and Lymphatics' role stressed in cardiovascular disease. Med World News Jan 21, 1966: 100-101.

ADDITIONAL CARDIAC BIBLIOGRAPHY:

INFLUENCES PRESENTLY UNCLASSIFIED

Beal MC: Viscerosomatic reflexes: A review. JAOA Dec 1985; 85: 786-801.

Blood HA: Manipulative management of hypertension. AAO Yearbook 1964; 189-195.

Burchett GB: Somatic manifestations of ischemic heart disease. Osteopathic Annals Sep 1976; 45-50.

Clymer DO: Effects of osteopathic manipulation on several different physiologic functions: Part III. JAOA Oct 1972; 72: 201-207.

Cox JM: Palpable musculoskeletal findings in coronary artery disease: Results of a double blind study. JAOA July 1983; 82: 832-836.

Fichera AP, Celander DR: Effect of osteopathic manipulative therapy on autonomic tone as evidenced by blood pressure changes and activity of the fibrinolytic system. JAOA Jun 1969; 68: 72-74.

Frymann V: In cardiac patients: Osteopathic manipulation held to aid heart function. Clinical Trends Osteopathic Medicine Mar-Apr 1976; 2:1, 5.

Johnson FE: Some observations on the use of osteopathic therapy in the care of patients with cardiac disease. JAOA May 1972; 71: 799-804.

Kellner A: Lipid and protein content of tissue fluid in normal and hyper-lipimic rabbits, in Symposium on Atherosclerosis. Washington DC, National Academy of Sciences National Research Council Publication, 1955, pp 42-49

Lymphatics role stressed in cardiovascular disease. Medical World News Jan 21, 1966: 100-101.

Malliani A: Evidence for a spinal sympathetic regulation of cardiovascular functions. Experentia 1970; 26): 965-966.

Mayerson HS: One aspect of role of lymphatic system in cardiovascular function in The Heart and Circulation: Vol I. (RC 681-AIN 3), pp 90-91.

Miller A: Effects of soft tissue manipulative therapy and factors regulating blood pressure. JAOA May 1967; 66: 990-991.

Miller AJ: The lymphatic system and cardiac disease (Chap. X), in Mayerson HS (ed) Proceedings of the Conference on Lymph and the Lymphatic System. CC Thomas, 1968.

Nicholas AS, et al: A Somatic component to myocardial infarction. British Medical Journal Jul 6, 1985; 291: 13-17.

Patriquin DA: Manipulation for the patient with myocardial infarction. Osteopathic Symposium Feb 1975; 16.

Reder RF: The role of the sympathetic nervous system in sudden cardiac death. Drug Therapy (Hospital) Jul 1978; 43-55.

Richmond WG: Influence of somatic manipulation in coronary artery disease evaluated by a controlled method. JAOA Jan 1942; 41: 217-225.

Rogers JL: The role of osteopathic manipulative therapy in the treatment of coronary heart disease. JAOA Sep 1976; 76: 21-31.

Stiles E: Congestive heart failure. Osteopathic Medicine Aug 1976; 76-78.

Stiles EG: Osteopathic approach to the hypertensive patient. Osteopathic Medicine Apr 1977; 44-45.

Stookey JR: OMT for angina. Osteopathic Symposium Mar 1975; 16-18.

Thomas PE: The role of the autonomic nervous system in arteriosclerosis. Osteopathic Annals Jan 1974; 12: 17-20.

Tilley M: The somatic component in heart disease. Osteopathic Annals May 1974; 30-43.

THE THORACOLUMBAR REGION AND CHAPMAN'S REFLEX INFLUENCES

Mannino JR: The application of neurologic reflexes to the treatment of hypertension. JAOA Dec 1979; 79(4): 225-231.

Comments on hypertension study. JAOA; 79(10): 607-608.

Value of manipulation unresolved by hypertensive study. JAOA; 79(11): 667-668.

THE CERVICAL REGION INFLUENCES

Johnson W: Palpatory findings in the cervicothoracic region: Variations in normotensive and hypertensive subjects, A preliminary report. JAOA Jan 1980; 79(5): 300-308.

CRANIAL CONCEPT INFLUENCES

Magoun HI Osteopathy in the Cranial Field. Kirksville MO, Journal Printing Co, 3rd ed, 1966, pp 114-115, 176, 179, 280.

Northup TL: Osteopathic cranial technique and its influence on hypertension. AAO Yearbook 1948: 70-77.

BEHAVIOR MODIFICATION INFLUENCE

Combined pharmacological and psychosocial therapies for hypertension discussed. Behavioral Medicine Sept 1980; 7(9): 3.

Relaxing hypertension in the long run. Emergency Medicine Jan 15, 1981; 177.

Wadden T, De La Torre C: Relaxation therapy as an adjunct treatment for essential hypertension. Journal of Family Practice 1980; 11(6): 901-903.

DIETARY CONSIDERATIONS

Hunt JC: The influence of diet on hypertension management. <u>Dialogues in Hypertension</u> 1980; IV: 37-47.
Silverberg DS: Treating hypertension with diet. <u>Consultant</u> Jul 1980; 115-120.

RISK CONSIDERATIONS

Finnerty FA: Hypertension: Current management, Part I, Selecting and evaluating the patient. <u>Consultant</u> Jan 1978; 163-168.
Thind G: Factors influencing hypertension prognosis and treatment. <u>Practical Cardiology</u> Apr 1980; 6(4): 31-39.
Klatsky AL: Alcohol and hypertension: Does drinking increase the risk? <u>Primary Cardiology</u> May 1978; 31-35, 64-65.

NOTES:

OSTEOPATHIC CONSIDERATIONS IN UPPER GI DISORDERS

"Manipulative therapy can play a major role in the management of the ulcer problem, both specifically and supportively, and it should be a routine and continuing feature of the emergency, maintenance, and follow-up care of the patient."[1]

I. INTRODUCTION

Along with backache and the common cold, gastrointestinal (GI) dysfunction is a very common cause for absence from work. Regardless of the etiology for the gastrointestinal upset, there will always be general and local as well as metabolic and cellular dysfunctions. Good therapeutic results from manipulation have been clinically reported by osteopathic physicians and supported for almost 100 years by patients who have received this distinctive manipulative treatment as a part of their total medical management.

Osteopathic manipulative treatment of patients with musculoskeletal dysfunction is understood by most individuals. The present understanding of pathophysiologic mechanisms and recent research in reflex neurophysiology has identified where and how osteopathic manipulation is also clinically effective in systemic dysfunction and disease. The "cause/effect approach" which these studies suggest should encourage the incorporation of directed manipulative care in treatment programs for patients with systemic disease and should stimulate more clinical research for documentation of the specific effects of manipulation in patients with gastrointestinal disease. Osteopathic manipulation is not given instead of medication nor are its effects upon the body's homeostatic mechanisms duplicated by the medications. Osteopathic manipulation directed toward improving the physiologic function of the patient and the use of pharmaceuticals directed mainly toward the disease work synergistically to encourage the patient's optimal ability to recover and to stay well.

II. PATHOPHYSIOLOGY

VISCEROSENSORY AND VISCEROMOTOR PATTERNS:

Pain patterns from viscerosomatic dysfunction are extremely important when performing a differential diagnosis on a patient with gastrointestinal (GI) complaints or when making clinical judgment of the severity of the underlying problem. Proper clinical analysis of these patterns requires a thorough understanding of both GI anatomy and neuroanatomy. Knowledge of the segmental innervation of GI organs and the location of the appropriately associated collateral sympathetic ganglion (see page 107) is vital for localizing the source of pain.

Pacinian corpuscles and free nerve endings are located in the wall of any given viscera. These receptors are activated by spasm or stretch; pain sensation is carried by visceral afferent fibers which travel a course similar to the corresponding splanchnic nerves.

True visceral pain carried by visceral afferent fibers often spills over into related right or left somatic segments in the back (depending upon which side the affected organ is on) and to the midline of the trunk (in organs derived from midline embryological structures).

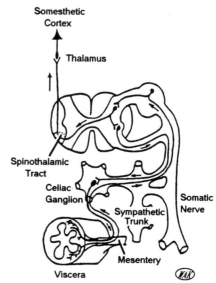

1. True visceral pain: This is early pain from irritation, stretching, contraction or exaggerated physiologic motor activity and dysfunction. It is midline pain, poorly localized and described as a vague, deep, diffuse burning ache.

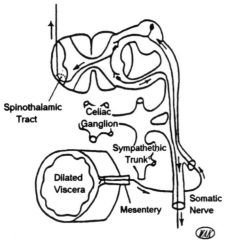

2. Viscerosensory pain often called viscerosomatic pain: This involves facilitated cord segments which permit visceral hypersympathicotonia as well as paraspinal somatic changes, joint somatic dysfunction, and dermatome hyperalgesia in somatic areas related to the viscera's sympathethic innervation.

All pain receptors which transmit impulses through visceral afferent fibers and the cerebrospinal tract are found within 2 cm of the gut and are stimulated by edema, pressure, torsion, traction, infiltration, bacterial toxins, enzymes, or friction. More specifically, they are found in the anterior and lateral parietal peritoneum, the lesser omentum, the mesentery, and the mesocolon.

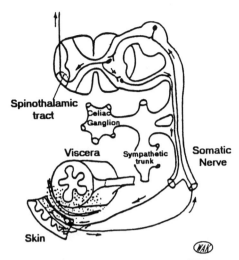

Spinothalamic tract

Celiac Ganglion

Viscera

Sympathetic trunk

Somatic Nerve

Skin

3. **Percutaneous Reflex of Morley:** This is direct transfer of inflammatory irritation from the viscera to the parietal peritoneum and abdominal wall without reflex through the visceral afferent nerve on a somatic afferent near the mesentary. It produces abdominal wall rigidity, pain, and rebound tenderness.

There are no receptors for pain in the visceral peritoneum; therefore the greater omentum and the spleen and its capsule are pain-insensitive structures. These structures produce awareness of pain only if they affect some adjacent, pain-sensitive structure. Visceral pain may become severe enough to spill over to areas of corresponding somatic segmental cerebrospinal distribution. Early in most disease processes, smooth muscle spasm or stretch will elicit visceral pain which is poorly localized and often described as gnawing, burning, or cramping. Sweating, nausea, vomiting, pallor, and a relentless attempt to squirm away from the pain is particularly characteristic of patients who are experiencing visceral pain. None of these common symptoms of visceral pain accompany somatic pain.

Somatic pain arises when the underlying visceral process progresses past the visceral serosa and stimulates adjacent somatic sensory nerves. Somatic pain is well-localized, asymmetric, and aggravated by jarring motions. Somatic pain may be added to the visceral pain pattern or it may overwhelm and mask it.

Phrenic pain (C3-5 referral area) occurs when either the hemi-diaphragm or Glisson's capsule of the liver is stimulated. Its somatic zone of referred pain is the ipsilateral shoulder cap. In 5% of patients, the fibers of the right phrenic nerve also reach the lesser omentum. In those people, stimulation of the lesser omentum would also produce phrenic type referred pain referral to the soma.

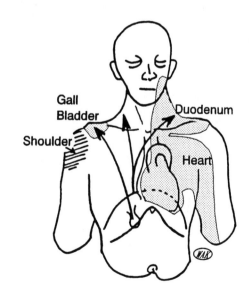

Gall Bladder

Duodenum

Shoulder

Heart

As a consequence of the spinal cord region becoming facilitated from increased and prolonged visceral afferent input, palpatory tissue changes and tenderness to palpation becomes evident in the segmental T5-9 paraspinal tissues, collateral ganglia and Chapman's reflex sites (page 232). Posteriorly, the small rotatores paraspinal muscles seem to be more frequently affected and their motion characteristics and the location of their dysfunction is a key to the source of the visceral dysfunction. They tend to exhibit the non-neutral type motion with a preference for backward bending and rotation and sidebending to the same side as the organ involved. While not contraindicated, high velocity, low amplitude (HVLA) OMT, is often found to be ineffective and is met with a rubbery resistance when applied to viscerosomatic dysfunction of this sort. This response should alert the clinician to look for an underlying visceral cause. If secondary somatic dysfunction is successfully treated with OMT, it often recurs; therefore, recurrent thoracic or rib somatic dysfunction without an apparent primary biomechanical cause should provoke a thorough examination for associated visceral organ dysfunction.

Common pain patterns for perforated and non-perforated upper abdominal problems were compiled by a group of physicians from the Mayo Clinic.[2] The following figures are illustrations adapted from that atlas.

TYPICAL PAIN PATTERN
PEPTIC ULCER

TYPICAL PAIN PATTERN
CHOLELITHIASIS WITH COLIC

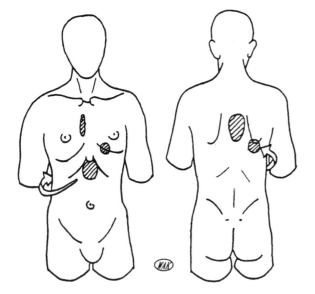

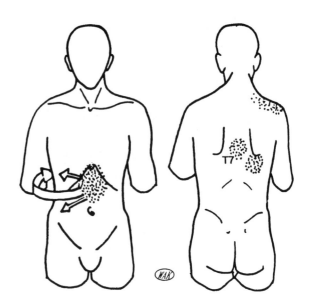

SYMPATHETICS:

The autonomic nervous system (ANS) innervates the viscera and most physiologists consider it soley an efferent system. Visceral afferent fibers report visceral dysfunction and they usually travel afferently along adjacent pathways as the corresponding efferent thoracic and lumbar sympathetic splanchnic nerves.

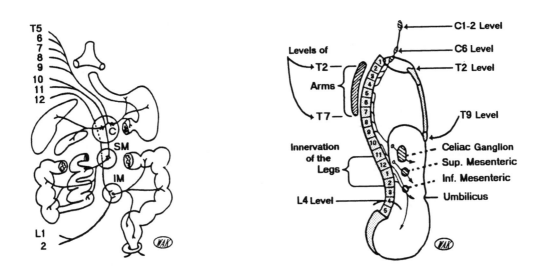

Somatic clues secondary to visceral dysfunction are mediated by visceral afferents to the cord and related somatic efferent fibers to the soma. These reflexes are called viscerosomatic reflexes.

These reflexes are responsible for much of the typical objective somatic pain patterns seen from visceral problems. They are also responsible for palpable Chapman's reflexes, and the characteristic paraspinal tissue texture changes related to facilitated cord segments T5-9 and T10-11. Visceral afferent activity is responsible for the early tissue changes palpable over the midline collateral sympathetic ganglia.

The sympathetic portion of the ANS has the unique ability to produce rapid and widespread organ and somatic changes required to meet stressful situations. Activation of one sympathetic fiber produces anywhere from four to forty post-ganglionic fiber activations. This is not always beneficial in dysfunction, illness, or disease where the patient has no need for the "fight or flight" function of the sympathetic system. Sodeman and Sodeman in <u>Pathologic Physiology: Mechanisms of Disease</u> state, "The adaptive protective reaction might be far more damaging to the individual than the noxious agent of the beginning dysfunction."[3] This is the situation occurring with prolonged sympathetic hyperactivity in GI dysfunction or disease.

Increased sympathetic tone decreases mucosal defenses against digestive acids and enzymes by producing vasoconstriction and alteration of the bicarbonate and mucous buffers. More patients develop inflammation or ulceration in the upper GI system from reduced mucosal defenses (from sympathicotonia) than from hyperacidity. Sympathetic activity also plays an important role in sphincter tone within the GI system. The normalization of facilitated segments and the associated sympathetic outflow from the T5-T11 region reduces gastrointestinal vasoconstriction and allows an increase in mucous secretion from Brunner's glands permitting homeostatic mechanisms to operate to protect mucous membranes.[4]

In diseased patients, prolonged hypersympathetic activity can initiate processes that are detrimental to survival. Gilsdorf and his group in 1965 reported in JAMA that cats with nonlethal pancreatitis would develop hemorrhagic necrotizing pancreatitis leading to the death of the animal when subjected to increased sympathetic stimulation; Block and others, writing in Surgical Gynecology and Obstetrics in 1954, indicated that ischemia changed nonlethal pancreatitis to lethal pancreatitis. From studying the world literature, Dr. Korr emphatically states, "In every disease process there is hypersympathetic activity; sustained sympathetic activity is a common factor in disease."

PARASYMPATHETICS:

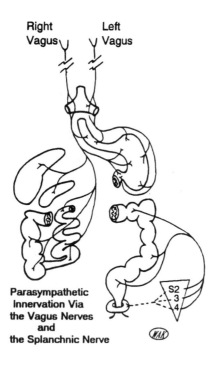

Right Vagus   Left Vagus

Parasympathetic Innervation Via the Vagus Nerves and the Splanchnic Nerve

S2 3 4

The parasympathetic portion of the ANS tends to dominate innervation of the viscera during "normal," long term, restful activity. In the upper GI tract, parasympathetic innervation is supplied by the vagus nerve (CN X) which exits the skull through the jugular foramen, which is formed by the joining of the jugular notch of the temporal and the jugular notch of the occipital bones. The left vagus supplies the greater curvature of the stomach and extends to the duodenum; the right vagus supplies the lesser curvature of the stomach, the small intestines, the right colon and the organs and glands up to the midtransverse colon.

Parasympathetic stimulation will increase the secretion rate of almost all gastrointestinal glands.[5]

The most inferior ganglion of the vagus nerve, the ganglion nodosum, extends into the cervical area and lies in fascias which are just anterior to the OA and AA joints. The vagus also has connections with the first two cervical somatic nerves which provide neurologic pathways for fibers carrying pain fibers from the posterior portion of the head (i.e. the occipital nerves). This connection may explain the occipital headaches which are often a part of the "subjective" symptomatology of a patient with upper GI or pulmonary disease, especially in upper GI viral dysfunctions or viral pneumonia.

This connection may also explain the nausea and vomiting that accompanies certain headaches and the palpatory clues found at the OA and C2 areas are related to dysfunction in viscera innervated by the vagus nerve. The parasympathetic system will also often produce symptoms of disease. Parasympathetic reflexes give the physician an explanation for many of the symptoms which are designated as nervous type or "functional disorders." These include hyperchlorhydria, nausea, hypermotility of the intestines, spastic colon, irritable bowel, bradycardia, asthma, hay fever, epiphoria, cough, hoarseness and excessive nasal discharge. The parasympathetic nervous system may also produce changes in tissues of its innervation, making that organ more susceptible to infection or chronic trophic change. It appears that all organs innervated by the vagus nerve are intimately bound together and capable of readily transmitting reflexes to and receiving reflexes from each other. This may be why the larynx is so often involved when there is a problem with some other part of the GI tract also innervated by cranial nerve X.[6]

LYMPHATICS:

The lymphatic system is absolutely necessary for good health and is even more important and frequently overworked during body dysfunction and disease. Extensive experimental studies in cats and dogs indicate that the lymphatic system must be able to increase its normal flow capacity by 4-5 times with some body stresses and in some chronic pathological syndromes such as congestive heart failure, up to 40 times its resting capacity. Because of these demands on its peak function, even a slight mechanical impedance of its lymphatic pathways or hindrance to the function of the diaphragm (which acts as its extrinsic pump) might greatly reduce the body's ability to recover from a disease process.

Lymph from the GI tract as well as all other organs and systems below the diaphragm drain from small lymphatic channels into the cisterna chyli. This is an irregular fibromuscular sac about the size of a cigarette, wedged between the aorta and the right crus of the diaphragm and just in front of the bodies of the

85

first two lumbar vertebrae. It also marks the start of the left lymphatic duct, called the thoracic duct.

The thoracic duct is about 18 inches long and extends from the cisterna chyli up through the fascias of the left thoracic inlet, into the neck for a distance of about 1 1/2 inches above the clavicle, arches over the pleura and apex of the left lung, and then passes back through the thoracic inlet to finally empty into the junction of the left internal jugular and left subclavian veins. The vital flow of lymph may be hindered by a poorly efficient, flattened diaphragm or by torsion of the fascias around the lymphatic channels located in the mesenteries or at the thoracic inlet. The first sign of terminal lymphatic drainage dysfunction in the abdomen may be a palpable fullness in the sub-xiphoid soft tissues.

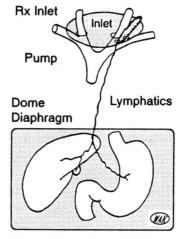

Upper Gastrointestinal Tract

Studies show that the incidence of pancreatitis is increased in gallbladder disease if their common lymphatic drainage route is compromised. Lymphatic drainage from the liver is increased greatly by minor pressure changes and so lymphatic drainage is greatly influenced by the depth of respirations and manipulative treatments (such as the liver pump) which create intermittent pressure charges.

SOMATIC SYSTEM:

Locating and correlating palpable changes in the musculoskeletal system are very helpful when considering a diagnosis of visceral disease. Reflex muscle spasm is often present in addition to segmental paraspinal somatic dysfunction, Chapman's reflexes and collateral ganglion tenderness. Guarding, rigidity and myofascial trigger points are all expressions of this phenomenon and all should be considered when performing a physical examination. Unless these areas are treated, pain patterns may be perpetuated. Travell reports, "Pain, which previously had responded to medical therapy for a duodenal ulcer, became unresponsive and persisted until trigger points in the abdominal musculature were found and inactivated."[7] Peptic ulcer disease has been found to be associated with abdominal myofascial trigger points which in turn continued to produce a somatic pain referral pattern similar to that originally produced by the visceral disturbance; in these patients, even after the ulcer healed, both the patient and physician are often misled to believe that a visceral problem remained. This is believed to be the case in postcholecystectomy syndrome where OMT commonly alleviates symptoms of gallbladder dysfunction and the typical gallbladder-type referred pain which remain even after surgical removal of the gallbladder.

III. THE PHILOSOPHY OF TREATMENT

The exact diagnosis is important when formulating specific medical and manipulative treatment and when predicting the prognosis for a patient with some type of disease process; however, from a functional standpoint, specific evaluation of the body's attempted homeostatic reactions to its dysfunction is often more useful than the specific visceral diagnosis when deciding where, how and what manipulative treatment to give. If the physician understands the general pathophysiology and responses of the upper GI tract to a disease process and can determine the responses of the patient to the dysfunction, manipulation can be beneficially administered even during the diagnostic work-up stages, to relax the patient and to support body homeostasis.

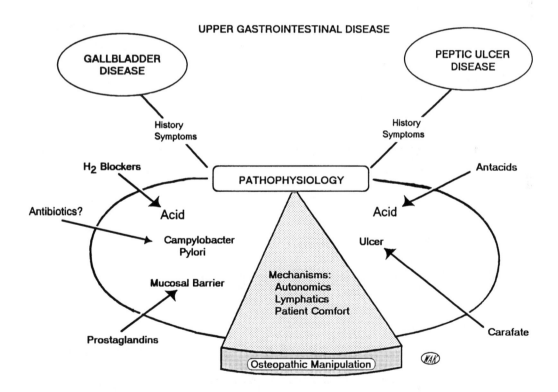

Therefore, the goal is not to diagnose and treat "joint dysfunction." The goal of treating patients in this manner involves administering rib raising and paraspinal inhibition for autonomic imbalance and reflex dysfunctions, improving circulatory and trophic factors, modifying fascial patterns which hinder lymphatic pathways and the pumps, and treating the base of the skull and upper cervical area to affect parasympathetic function. If specific joint somatic dysfunction is palpable it should be diagnosed and treated appropriately, because it represents a somatic contribution to the maintenance of the facilitated segments of the cord and thus hinders the viscera by its promotion of sympathetic hyperactivity, termed sympathicotonia.

It is not unusual to see patients suffering from pain and cramping discomfort due to GI dysfunction of many types, waiting uncomfortably for 1-3 days while the "specific diagnosis" is being obtained through multiple test procedures. Manipulative treatment for those patients could be started early. This would not interfere with the diagnosis in any way, once the search for an organic etiology was planned and in progress; in fact, the responses of the musculoskeletal system may help guide a more economical or complete approach to the diagnosis. It would make the patient more comfortable by beginning normalization of altered physiologic processes at a connective tissue or cellular level. Manipulative treatment would most likely reduce the amount of pain medication required for patient comfort and would help prepare the patient's body for better acceptance, distribution and utilization of any specific medications prescribed once the pathologic diagnosis is secured. If the process was functional, then often the "negative" work-up for organic structural causes will be accompanied by a patient who no longer has complaints.

Osteopathic manipulation for a patient with systemic disease is primarily directed toward balancing autonomic activity and improving lymphatic flow. This type of treatment should relieve, improve and enhance the patient's own abilities:

o to improve visceral response to stress
o to relieve congestion
o to improve circulation
o to enhance the removal of waste products from the tissues
o to improve cardiac output
o to improve oxygenation and nutrition at a cellular level
o to enhance resistance to infection
o to enhance more predictable tissue levels and patient response to specific
      medications
o to enhance relaxation and comfort of the patient during diagnostic
      procedures and any specific treatment program

IV. OSTEOPATHIC TREATMENT FOR PATIENT WITH UPPER GI DYSFUNCTION

LYMPHATICS AND FASCIAS:

The visceral organs are suspended from the dorsal surface of the abdominal cavity by mesenteries. Through these connective tissue pathways pass the arterial blood supply, the venous and lymphatic drainage vessels, and the sympathetic, parasympathetic and visceral afferent nerves of the viscera.

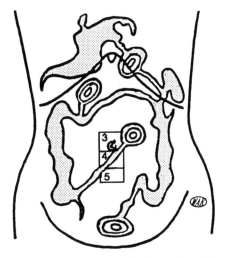

Location of Mesenteric Attachments

The most important mesentery to the osteopathic physician who is treating upper GI dysfunction is the mesentery for attachment of the small intestines. This mesentery can be located in the patient by constructing an imaginary line from 1 inch to the left and 1 inch above the umbilicus to a point in the lower right quadrant of the abdomen just anterior to the right sacroiliac joint. Thirty feet of intestines are attached to this six-inch mesenteric base.

A manipulative technique to reduce congestion and improve circulation to the small intestines is called a "mesenteric lift" and is helpful in freeing lymphatic pathways from the small intestines. The small intestines usually lie in the suprapubic and lower left abdominal quadrants. This ventral abdominal technique for the small intestines is performed by carefully lifting them upward and to the right side of the abdomen while using the patient's respiratory force for activation (see page 227). The patient's respiratory force is activated by having the patient breathe in and hold the breath until air hunger occurs. The physician should be sensitive to the tissue response under the palpating fingers and keep the patient comfortable while providing a gentle encouragement to the tissues being treated. About the time the patient needs to take a breath, the physician will feel a mesenteric release (although occasionally 2-3 breath cycles will be required before a release is palpated). Visceral manipulation using release techniques for each upper GI organ has been described in detail by Jean-Pierre Barral, D.O.,[8] and may be employed to help maximize visceral function.

The fascial pattern of the thoracic inlet and the inferior thoracic outlet must also be evaluated. These fascial areas are treated as indicated and the diaphragm must be well domed. "Domed" means that both leaves of the relaxed diaphragm are optimally concave inferiorly (convex superiorly) and that they work symmetrically during respiration. Treatment of a dysfunction of the thoracoabdominal diaphragm might include soft tissue to the paraspinal muscles and quadratus lumborum as well as direct or indirect fascial treatment directed at the diaphragmatic attachments--the thoracolumbar junction, the lower six ribs, and/or the sternum.

SYMPATHETICS:

Any stress or dys-function of the upper GI tract causes a bar-rage of visceral affer-ent impulses to bom-bard the cord. Vis-ceral afferents from the upper GI tract and small intestines travel first through the celiac or superior mesenteric collateral ganglia. They then travel through the chain ganglia to cord levels T5 to T11.[9]

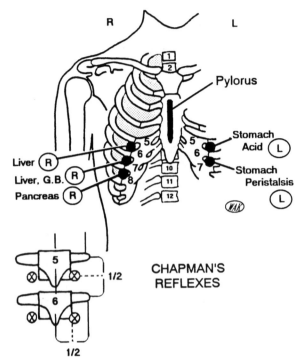

Since these impulses tend to travel the same pathways as corresponding sympathetic efferents, any resultant facilitated segments are more likely to be at the levels of sympathetic innervation to the organ in trouble. Studies confirm that somatic palpatory clues to upper GI and small intestinal dysfunction occur in the paraspinal somatic tissues from T5 to T11.

Chapman's system of anterior and posterior myofascial tender points related to specific visceral dysfunction are particularly helpful in diagnosis of GI dysfunc-tion.[10] They are considered to be produced by viscerosomatic reflexes which generally fit a sympathetic reflex pattern.

Charts for the entire Chapman system of anterior and posterior myofascial points can be obtained[11] and are reproduced in diagrams on pages 232 and 233. The anterior points are most useful as indicators of dysfunction because they are easily located and are more sensitive to light palpation. They correlate well with final hospital diagnoses.[12] The posterior points are less tender; therefore, they are less often used as diagnostic clues. Some physicians use the posterior

90

points for localized soft tissue treatment in an attempt to influence a specific organ's autonomic balance.

The above knowledge helps a physician diagnose and plan manipulative treatment for upper GI disease and dysfunction. Treatment to normalize sympathetic hyperactivity is clinically effective and may be administered in several different areas including the sementally associated vertebrae (facilitated segments), the ribs (sympathetic chain ganglia), the specific collateral ganglion, and the Chapman's reflex tender points.

Any treatment to the sympathetic ganglia will initially stimulate sympathetic activity to the organs of sympathetic innervation, but this effect is localized near the segments treated and is short-lived. The lasting effect is believed to be produced through stimulation of the long very slow sympathetic fibers, which cause inhibition of sympathetic outflow in the areas treated. This reaction is centrally mediated and is longer acting. It serves to improve blood flow and maximize homeostasis including mucosal barriers to areas of the GI system sharing the same segmental distribution.

o .. RIB RAISING: The most common manipulative method to modify sympathetic activity utilizes rib raising techniques (page 195) to the appropriate rib areas, i.e. T5-T11 for the upper GI tract and small intestines. Since the chain ganglia of the sympathetics lie in the fascias over the heads of the ribs, rib raising produces the reflexes which clinically normalize sympathetic activity. This technique can be administered with the patient in the supine, lateral recumbent or sitting position. Treatment only needs to be long enough for the physician to sense palpable tissue change. This may take a few seconds to a few minutes.

It is known that spinal impulses passing through a facilitated area of the spinal cord will produce bursts of sympathetic activity to the viscera innervated by those segments. For this reason, treatment of segmental spinal somatic dysfunctions related to areas of suspected facilitated cord segments often precedes manipulative techniques to other tissues in other areas.

O .. VENTRAL ABDOMINAL INHIBITION: Treatment by ventral abdominal inhibition to the appropriate collateral sympathetic ganglia (page 200) until tissue change is palpable is also considered to reduce sympathetic hyperactivity of their respective spinal levels. It is known that the collateral ganglia are able to provide some regional control of the viscera without relay to the central nervous system and are not "just switching stations" for autonomic activity.

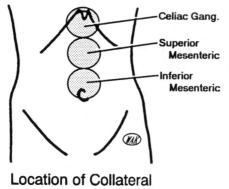

Location of Collateral
Sympathetic Ganglia

These ganglia are located in the midline of the abdomen--anterior to the abdominal aorta and between the xiphoid process and the umbilicus. The celiac ganglion is associated with T5-9; the superior mesenteric ganglion with T10-11; and the inferior mesenteric ganglion with T12-L2. The first two named ganglia are often involved in upper GI disorders while the inferior mesenteric ganglion is involved in lower GI and pelvic problems.

O .. CHAPMAN'S MYOFASCIAL POINTS: (See pages 232 and 233) Sympathetic hyperactivity can also be treated by manipulation of posterior Chapman's reflex points. The anterior Chapman's points are easily accessible and more tender to manipulation so are used for diagnosis. Memorize the common anterior Chapman's points related to the gastrointestinal system. When performing a physical examination, these clues to visceral dysfunction can be checked in just a few seconds. These ganglioform reflex points are believed to be produced in the deep myofascial tissues by viscersomatic reflexes resulting in increased hypersympathetic. If one or more are tender to palpation, ask specific questions related organ's dysfunction and correlate this with findings from palpation of the collateral sympathetic ganglia and related paraspinal tissues. To treat the posterior points related to the upper GI tract and small intestines, circular soft tissue pressure of moderate intensity is administered between the proper intertransverse processes until the points disappear. Posterior Chapman's points related to the upper GI system in the intertransverse spaces will usually correlate with tender anterior Chapman's points located in the respective ipsilateral intercostal spaces.

PARASYMPATHETIC SYSTEM:

Beneficial treatment to improve parasympathetic innervation to the upper GI tract is directed primarily toward removing joint somatic dysfunction of the cervical spine (especially in the area of the OA and AA joints), treating the soft tissues of the suboccipital area and utilizing condylar decompression techniques to relieve fascial tensions around the ganglion nodosum and the vagal trunks. If the physician is trained in cranial treatment techniques, treating somatic dysfunctions of the occipitomastoid suture area will release tensions felt to affect the vagal nerve as it exits the skull through the jugular foramen. This treatment is also effective in helping to relieve tensions associated with suboccipital and occipital headaches which often accompany GI disturbances.

VI. SUMMARY

It has been shown that removal of musculoskeletal dysfunction may alter associated, secondary visceral dysfunction; however, if the musculoskeletal etiology remains too long, the reflex pathway seems to be "learned by the cord," so that the dysfunction of the viscera may be reestablished even after the somatic dysfunction is removed. Patterson hypothesizes that this may be a basis for a patient's predisposition to chronic disease and may indicate evidence supporting early osteopathic manipulation as a means of preventing diseases as well as a means of supporting a body that has disease.

Osteopathic manipulation provides an additional and synergistic approach to the usual medical treatment of GI disease and dysfunction. No matter how effective medicines become, drug specificity and sophistication does not excuse an osteopathic physician from the responsibility of supporting the patient's own defenses. Intelligent, physician-directed manipulation provides this support for the patient by enhancing the self-regulatory mechanisms of the body unit using OMT to improve the body's structure and function.

REFERENCES:

1. Strong WB: Disorders of the digestive system, in Hoag JM (ed) Osteopathic Medicine. New York, McGraw-Hill, 1969, ch 38, p 573.
2. Smith LA et al An Atlas of Pain Patterns: Sites and Behavior of Pain in Certain Common Diseases of the Upper Abdomen. Springfield IL, CC Thomas, 1961.
3. Sodeman WA, Sodeman TM Pathologic Physiology: Mechanisms of Disease. Philadelphia, WB Saunders, 6th ed, 1979.
4. Strong WB: Disorders of the digestive system, in Hoag JM (ed) Osteopathic Medicine. New York, McGraw-Hill, 1969, ch 38, p 573.
5. Pottenger FM Symptoms of Visceral Disease. St Louis, CV Mosby Co, 1953, 7th ed, 262.
6. Op cit pp 211-215.
7. Travell JG, Simons DG Myofascial Pain and Dysfunction: A Trigger Point Manual. Baltimore, Williams & Wilkins, 1983, p 674.
8. Barral JP, Mercier P Visceral Manipulation. Seattle WA, Eastland Press, 1988.
9. Beal MC: Viscerosomatic reflexes: A review. JAOA Dec 198;85:786-801.
10. Owens C An Endocrine Interpretation of Chapman's Reflexes. Carmel CA, 1963.
11. Contact the Department of Osteopathic Theory and Methods at the Kirksville College of Osteopathic Medicine, 800 West Jefferson Street, Kirksville, Mo. 63501
12. Byrnes TR, Kuchera ML, Guffey JM, Steele KM, Beatty DR, Haman JL, Lockwood MD: Correlation of palpatory findings with visceral diagnoses. JAOA 92(9): 1177, Sept 1992.

OSTEOPATHIC MANIPULATION OF A PATIENT WITH
UPPER GASTROINTESTINAL DYSFUNCTION

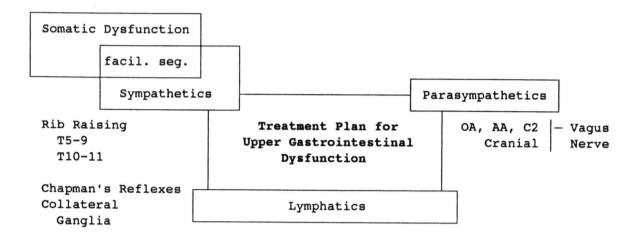

Cervicals C3-5 (Phrenic Nerve)
Thoracolumbar Junction (Diaphragm Attachment)

Somatic Dysfunction

facil. seg.

Sympathetics

Rib Raising
  T5-9
  T10-11

Chapman's Reflexes
Collateral
  Ganglia

Treatment Plan for
Upper Gastrointestinal
Dysfunction

Parasympathetics

OA, AA, C2 — Vagus
Cranial   Nerve

Lymphatics

Thoracic Inlets
 Abdominal Diaphragm
 Effleurage
 Lymphatic Pumps
 Mesenteric OMT (Ventral Abdominal Techniques)

SYMPATHETIC (PATHO)PHYSIOLOGY

↑ Tone:
1. ↑ Vascular Tone → ↓ O_2 and Nutrients to tissues
   → ↑ Mucosal Sensitivity to H^+ Concentration and Alters
   the Mucosal Barrier
2. Relaxation of Gallbladder and Ducts
3. ↓ Peristalsis → Constipation

LYMPHATIC (PATHO)PHYSIOLOGY

Impaired Lymph Flow:
1. ↑ Tissue Congestion and Impaired Nutrient Absorption from
   the Bowel
2. ↑ Risk of Pancreatic Complications in Gallbladder
   Disease/Dysfunction

PARASYMPATHETIC (PATHO)PHYSIOLOGY

↑ Tone:
1. ↑ Acid Secretion
2. Contraction of Gallbladder and Ducts
3. Peristalsis → Diarrhea

94

OSTEOPATHIC CONSIDERATIONS IN LOWER BOWEL DISORDERS

I. INTRODUCTION

Beginning cellular and organ dysfunctions associated with disturbed metabolism, congested tissues, cloudy swelling, lactic acid accumulation and tissue acidosis are reversible with early treatment. Visceral irritation and disease increase visceral afferent nerve activity and are often associated with hypersympathetic bombardment of the associated organs. Sympathetic nerve impulses may protect the body from external dangers but when they remain hyperactive, due to cord facilitation, they become a roadblock to rapid healing and restoration of health and can even produce potentially lethal conditions. Hypersympathetic activity is present in post-surgical patients and all patients with systemic diseases.

The rate of healing of body tissues is dependent upon the ability of the body to remove waste products from the tissues and to deliver oxygen and other nutrients to the area of tissue dysfunction, injury, or the site of a surgical intervention. This "is built in" to the body as self-regulating mechanisms which in turn require good arterial, venous and lymphatic circulation, as well as a good nerve supply. These prerequisites of the self-regulating mechanisms depend upon good circulation and accurate reports from visceral afferent nerves.

Hypoperfusion results in low tissue resistance to infection and when infected, these tissues remain infected longer than tissues with good perfusion and nutrition. Studies by Niinikoski (1980) reveal that white blood cells selectively kill bacteria by using superoxide and that "any treatment that augments the local oxygen supply to the tissues and helps to avoid hypoperfusion increases the rate of healing and decreases the susceptibility to infection." Han and McKay concluded from experimentation involving animal inoculations of *staphylococcal* bacteria that "even small increases in oxygen to a tissue resulted in a relative large increase in its resistance to infection and greatly increased its ability to recover from the infection."

Osteopathic manipulative treatment in bowel disease and bowel dysfunction is often directed toward and related to improving blood and lymphatic flow and balancing the autonomic impulses to and from the bowel. Effective osteopathic treatment improves the circulation and oxygenation of the tissues. When performing or ordering manipulative treatment for lower GI diseases, certain functional anatomical and neurologic peculiarities of the colon must be kept in mind.

II. PATHOPHYSIOLOGY

SYMPATHETICS:

Sympathetic hyperactivity reflecting a disease process is usually associated with facilitated segments T10-T11 when the right half of the colon is involved and facilitation of T12-L2 when the left half of the colon is involved. Disorders of the colon usually produce viscerosomatic reflexes which increase thoracolumbar paraspinal muscle tension and produce pain in T10-11 or T12-L2 areas of the spine.

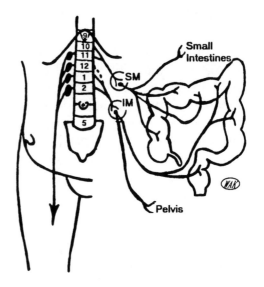

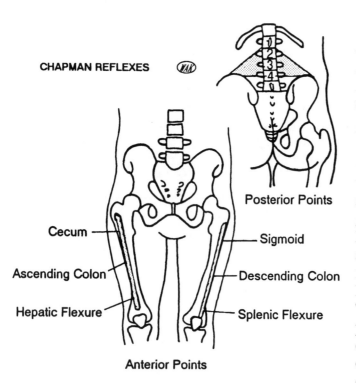

CHAPMAN REFLEXES

Posterior Points

Cecum

Ascending Colon

Hepatic Flexure

Sigmoid

Descending Colon

Splenic Flexure

Anterior Points

Sympathetic hyperactivity is also believed to be indicated by viscerosomatic myofascial tender points called Chapman's points.[1] This myofascial system of diagnosis and treatment is attributed to Frank Chapman, D.O. The anterior Chapman's points are helpful clues to colon dysfunction and are found as tender, palpable fascial ganglioform nodulations on the lateral side of the thighs in the anterior half of the iliotibial bands from the greater trochanters to the lateral epicondyles of the femur. These areas become tender to light pressure with most colon dysfunction; however, it has been clinically observed that some colon cancers may not produce

Chapman's reflexes though it is not known exactly why this is true. It is theorized that tissue inflammation and/or irritation is required to initiate these reflexes through the visceral afferent and sympathetic systems.

With diseases of the colon, the inferior collateral sympathetic ganglion, located in the midline of the abdomen and just above the umbilicus, is often palpable and tender. This palpatory change is also believed to indicate sympathetic hyperactivity to the colon as a result of visceral afferent bombardment with its influence upon facilitation of related cord segments.

The collateral ganglia in the midline of the abdomen have self-contained mechanisms which can attempt control and reaction to regional visceral dysfunction; therefore, they are capable of controlling function locally without reporting to the spinal cord.

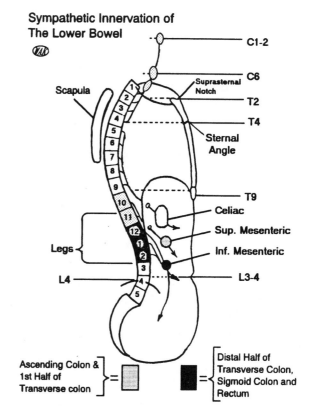

Sympathetic Innervation of The Lower Bowel

Ascending Colon & 1st Half of Transverse colon $=$

Distal Half of Transverse Colon, Sigmoid Colon and Rectum $=$

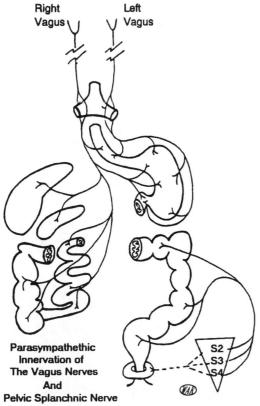

Parasympathethic Innervation of The Vagus Nerves And Pelvic Splanchnic Nerve

Sympathetic hyperactivity of the lower GI system is associated with findings and symptoms of ileus, constipation, abdominal distention and flatulence.

PARASYMPATHETICS:

Manipulative techniques to normalize parasympathetic activity to the colon may be especially useful in the care of patients with colitis, Crohn's disease, irritable bowel syndrome, or idiopathic diarrhea. The vagus nerve provides parasympathetic innervation to the right side of the colon.

The left vagal innervation extends only to the greater curvature of the stomach and the pyloric area of the GI tract. The right vagus nerve also innervates the upper GI tract, including the lesser curvature of the stomach, the liver and gall bladder and then continues on to innervate all of the small intestines and the right half of the colon. The pelvic splanchnic nerves with their origin from cord segments S2,3,4, supply the parasympathetic innervation of the left half of the colon and the pelvis.

This split in parasympathetic innervation must be kept in mind when looking for somatic dysfunction which could have an affect on the right or the left half of the colon.

Parasympathetic hyperactivity in the lower GI system increases bowel motility and glandular secretions and is associated with diarrhea. Hypoactivity of the parasympathetic system results in the opposite manifestations of bowel function, namely decreased bowel motility and glandular secretion as well as constipation. When there is hyperactivity of both the parasympathetic and the sympathetic systems to the bowel the functional disorder tends to manifest as an irritable bowel syndrome. (See Irritable Bowel Syndrome, page 109.)

LYMPHATICS:

With dysfunction of the tissues of the colon there are cellular and tissue metabolic changes which lead to increased interstitial fluids and tissue congestion. The result is accumulation of waste products, reduced oxygenation and decreased nutrition to the cells. These changes increase the colon's susceptibility to inflammation and infection and increases its healing time when stressed. Congestion also increases the likelihood of fibrosis with increased scarring in the healing process. Fibrosis can worsen the prognosis in patients with colitis or Crohn's disease.

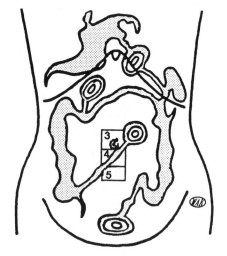

Location of Mesenteric Attachments

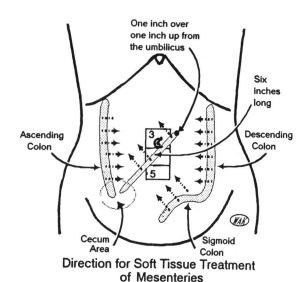

Direction for Soft Tissue Treatment of Mesenteries

Vessels and nerves to and from the intestines must travel in mesenteries. Though these mesenteries are broad, the very thin walls of the lymphatic and venous channels are vulnerable to pressure from surrounding edematous tissues. Canine studies indicate that tissue congestion interferes with the effective medical treatment of disease processes.[2]

In these studies there was uneven distribution and accumulation of the active drug in the dogs' tissues and the drug's by-products accumulated in the congested tissues; often the tissues which needed the active component the most were the tissues that got the least concentration.

According to Sam Threefoot, M.D., director of the New Orleans Research Institute, "When lymphatic flood channels fail to function because of anatomical fault or abnormal physiologic mechanisms, therapy is impeded."[3]

Because the interstitial fluids from a congested colon drain through the thoracic duct, any restriction of the lymphatic pathways to the duct, the fascias through which the duct passes, or the fascias at the thoracic inlet would be associated with increased tissue congestion. Thoracic diaphragm function should be ascertained because of its importance in moving both venous and lymphatic fluids. The ability of the pelvic diaphragm to passively and synchronously move with the abdominal diaphragm should also be considered when treating conditions associated with abdominopelvic congestion.

It is possible that patients with disease processes or prior surgery involving the lower sigmoid, rectum, and anal areas will have asymmetry or spasm of the pelvic diaphragm. The pelvic diaphragm is a funnel-shaped muscle attaching to the lateral walls of the true pelvis and angling inferiorly and medially to attach to the urogenital diaphragm and the midline structures of the urogenital and anal triangles. There are right and left leaves of the pelvic diaphragm.

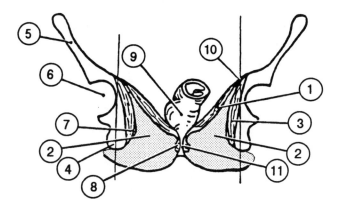

1. Pelvic Diaphragm
2. Ischiorectal Fossa
3. Obturator Internus Muscle
4. Ischial Tuberosity
5. Iliacus (Bone)
6. Acetabulum
7. Alcock's Canal (Pudendal Canal)
8. External Anal Sphincter
9. Rectum
10. Tendinous Arch of Obturator Internus Fascia
11. Anal Canal

99

The spaces below the pelvic diaphragm and between the diaphragm and the structures on the lateral walls of the true pelvis are filled with fat and are called the ischiorectal fossae. The pelvic diaphragm is innervated by the pudendal nerve originating from sacral roots S2,3,4. As mentioned earlier, these same cord segments provide the origin for the pelvic splanchnic nerves which supply the parasympathetic innervation to the left half of the colon, pelvis, and perineum. The pelvic diaphragm works most effectively when it is relaxed and can work passively and synchronously with the abdominal diaphragm.

Tension of the pelvic diaphragm is diagnosed by gently but firmly inserting the extended fingers of one hand into the lateral margin of one ischiorectal fossa, along the lateral side of the rectal triangle of the perineum. The same examination is carried out on the other side and the tensions of the muscle on the two sides are compared. An indication of the pelvic diaphragm tension could also be obtained during the performance of the usual rectal or vaginal examination. OMT to this region is described on page 216.

VISCEROSENSORY AND VISCEROMOTOR PATTERNS

The general principles listed in the previous chapter (Osteopathic Considerations in Upper GI Disorders) are also pertinent for the lower bowel.

SOMATIC

It is well documented that severe insult, such as a vertebral fracture, to thoracolumbar segmental levels will cause a somatovisceral reflex resulting in paralytic ileus. Travell and Simons report[4] several other visceral symptoms resulting from abdominal myofascial trigger points including diarrhea, vomiting, belching, food intolerance, and colic in the infant or excessive burping in an adult.

The somatic component of the viscerosomatic reflex that takes place because of the handling of the bowel during some surgeries is capable of initiating a secondary somatovisceral reflex which results in and maintains a paralytic post-operative ileus. (See study of effects of osteopathic manipulation in prevention and treatment of post-op ileus pages 103.) Treatment of the somatic component alleviates the symptoms of the resulting visceral dysfunction.

III. OSTEOPATHIC MANIPULATIVE TREATMENT OF COLON DYSFUNCTION

SUGGESTED PROTOCOL FOR PROVIDING OSTEOPATHIC MANIPULATIVE TREATMENT TO POST-OPERATIVE PATIENTS:

ADMINISTRATION IN GENERAL:

This protocol is especially useful in treatment of patients who have had abdominopelvic surgery. Optimum treatment frequency is three times a day until bowel sounds are heard regularly. Osteopathic manipulative technique and dosage must be modified depending upon the surgical site, placement of drainage tubes and location of incision and dressings.

STAGE I:

In the immediate post-operative period there are unequilibrated hemodynamics and electrolyte imbalance. Bowel sounds are very poor or absent on auscultation. There is shallow breathing from neuromuscular splinting. Palpation reveals significant reflex hypertonicity of paraspinal muscles from surgical interruption of associated dermatome and myotome segments while viscerosomatic reflexes from the surgical and manual irritation of the viscera also contribute to the paraspinal hypertonicity.

TREATMENT:

A. Gentle inhibition of hypertonic paravertebral muscles to point of tissue relaxation (2-5 minutes total time)
B. Gentle inhibition of hypertonic paravertebral muscles in thoracic region. This is most effectively directed toward spinal segments which are associated with the surgical site via supplying sympathetic innervation to the involved viscera.
C. Indirect method fascial release manipulation of the diaphragm, thoracic inlet and mid-cervical spine

STAGE II:

In this stage, there is less reflex neuromuscular splinting. Hemodynamics and electrolytes are near normal. Bowel sounds are present. The patient may be taking oral fluids. The breathing pattern has improved.

101

TREATMENT:

    A.   Apply inhibition to paravertebral muscles, especially at the paravertebral segments related to the sympathetic innervation of viscera involved in the area of surgery. Treat the segments until there is tissue change under the treating fingers
    B.   Rib raising each side (1-3 minutes)
    C.   Indirect method fascial release to thoracic and sternal region myofascial tissues
    D.   Indirect method fascial release to tissues near surgical site
    E.   Inhibition of cervical paravertebral areas as indicated by palpatory evaluation of the patient

STAGE III.

In this stage the patient is ambulating fairly well. Oral intake is improving. There is minimal reflex neuromuscular splinting.

TREATMENT:

    A.   Inhibition of paravertebral muscles at paravertebral segments associated with surgery (1-3 minutes)
    B.   Specific mobilization of segmental vertebral units or regions as indicated
    C.   Pectoral traction with modified classic lymphatic pump or pedal pump as possible and determined by evaluation of the patient (2 minutes as tolerated)

FOR OPTIMAL TREATMENT:

Add bilateral condylar decompression and CV4 treatment. This is a significant benefit to patients at all post-operative stages. Providing the CV4 treatment in these patients is limited only by the physician's ability to use it properly.

Abdominal mesenteric lift techniques help to decongest the colon and may be used when no abscess, abdominal aneurysm or acute infection is present in the area of treatment. Lymph flow is encouraged by appropriate lymphatic pumps (intermittent chest pressure, pectoralis lift or by utilizing a rocking motion of the abdominal contents through production of intermittent cephalad pressure through the lower extremities). See page 227 for ventral abdominal techniques and page 218 for lymphatic pumps. Visceral manipulations for each lower GI structure and pelvic organ have also been described in detail by Barral[5] and may be employed to maximize visceral function.

ILEUS PREVENTION TREATMENT:

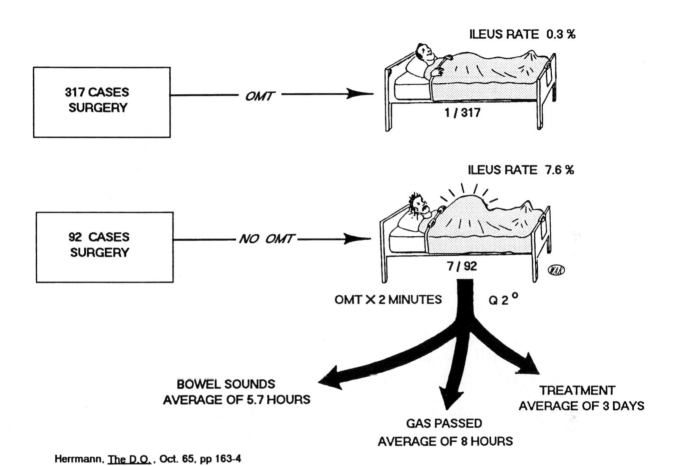

ILEUS RATE 0.3 %

317 CASES
SURGERY

OMT

1 / 317

ILEUS RATE 7.6 %

92 CASES
SURGERY

NO OMT

7 / 92

OMT X 2 MINUTES   Q 2°

BOWEL SOUNDS
AVERAGE OF 5.7 HOURS

GAS PASSED
AVERAGE OF 8 HOURS

TREATMENT
AVERAGE OF 3 DAYS

Herrmann, The D.O., Oct. 65, pp 163-4

The above ileus prevention study[6] demonstrates the general importance and efficacy of osteopathic manipulative treatment in interrupting inappropriate viscerosomatic-somatovisceral cycles.

SUPPORTIVE MANIPULATION FOR PATIENTS WITH SPECIFIC FUNCTIONAL PROBLEMS AND COMPLAINTS:

PATIENTS WITH SYMPATHETIC DOMINANT COMPLAINTS: constipation, abdominal pain, flatulence, and distention.

In these patients the physician should palpate the iliotibial bands looking for diagnostic anterior Chapman points which might be related to colon irritation. The lumbothoracic and the lumbosacral areas are then relaxed with kneading and stretching soft tissue treatment. This addresses the important sympathetic levels while simultaneously relaxing the posterior attachments of the abdominal diaphragm. It also accomplishes treatment of the posterior Chapman points. The posterior Chapman points for the colon are located in a triangular area on each side of the lumbar spine. This area can be outlined (see page 96) by drawing an imaginary line from the crest of each ilium to the spine, then passing up the spine to the superior level of L2, and then connecting that point with the crest of the ilium again. Chapman found that light circular pressure or kneading to the triangular posterior Chapman area in the lumbar paraspinal tissues or light circular pressure and soft tissue to the iliotibial bands greatly reduces detrimental sympathetic outflow to the colon.

Hypersympathetic activity to the right colon is effectively reduced by rib raising in the T10-12 area and by paraspinal soft tissue techniques administered to the T12-L2 area of the spine. With the patient in the supine position, the midline of the abdomen between the xiphoid process and the umbilicus is palpated for tenderness, especially just above the umbilicus over the inferior mesenteric ganglion. If it is palpable and tender, carefully controlled inhibitory pressure is applied until a palpable relaxation of the tissues occurs in that area. It is clinically observed that manipulative treatments directed toward reducing sympathetic outflow reduce the pain experienced by patients with colon dysfunction. Manipulative treatment in the form of paraspinal inhibition to the thoracolumbar area also initiates bowel activity in patients with ileus and rapidly diminishes abdominal bloating.

PATIENTS WITH PARASYMPATHETIC DOMINANT COMPLAINTS: headache, nausea, vomiting, diarrhea, cramps or pain from the GI tract.

When associated with right-sided colon dysfunction, examination and manipulation are usually directed to the OA, AA, and occipitomastoid suture areas. More tissue dysfunction would be expected in the right suboccipital area because the right vagus nerve innervates the right colon. The right and left ganglia nodosum of the vagus lie in the fascial tissues just anterior to the OA and AA joints. These ganglia lie in and just below the jugular foramina of the skull. These areas should be examined for fascial tension or specific joint somatic dysfunction; the motion pattern and mobility of the cranium should also be determined. Condylar decompression and cranial techniques to ensure symmetry of motion in the occipitotemporal region (if the physician is trained in cranial manipulation) is effective treatment in a patient expressing symptoms related to the parasympathetic system. While in the area, the physician may as well palpate for somatic dysfunction of C3-5, because this area influences the phrenic nerve and function of the abdominal diaphragm.

When associated with left-sided colon dysfunction or pain, diagnose and manipulate somatic dysfunction of the sacrum, innominates, and lumbosacral regions. It is particularly important to check for unilateral sacral shear somatic dysfunction and the ability of the sacrum to passively rock about its involuntary superior transverse axis (the respiratory axis) between the innominates.

PATIENTS WITH OTHER RELATED COMPLAINTS: In all diseases of the colon, fatigue, constipation, diarrhea, pain and cramps may be related to lymphatic congestion of the colon.

The first step toward increasing lymphatic drainage from the colon is to check for fascial torsions and joint somatic dysfunction at the thoracic inlet. This includes examination of ribs 1 and 2, the first four thoracic vertebrae and the manubrium of the sternum. Any joint or fascial somatic dysfunction related to these tissues should be treated.

The patient may then be turned to the lateral recumbent position and given soft tissue treatment to relax the tissues of the lumbosacral junction. L1,2,3, is the area of the spinal attachment of the diaphragm and must be relaxed before the diaphragm can be redomed. The abdominal diaphragm also attaches to the lower 6 ribs and the xiphoid process. The diaphragm may be redomed with direct or indirect fascial techniques. It must be functioning properly in order to provide the effective pressure gradients needed to "pump" lymph from the abdomen to the thorax.

The pelvic diaphragm should be palpated and if treatment is indicated it can be accomplished by using an ischiorectal fossa technique (see page 216). Relaxation of the pelvic diaphragm through ischiorectal fossa techniques (or through transvaginal and anal digital inhibition treatment) helps to relieve congestion and pain originating in the pelvis and also relieves perineural edema of the pelvic parasympathetic nerves or the somatic pudendal nerve (both having their origin from nerve roots S2,3,4).

IV. SUMMARY

Osteopathic manipulation is physiologic treatment of a patient that may be directed toward systemic dysfunction and/or the body's response to a disease process. It is the condition of the body itself which determines whether, how efficiently and how completely a person will recover from a surgery, a systemic disease or an infective process. The development and the use of more powerful and specific drugs as a means of improving a patient's recovery will have varying effects depending upon the physician's ability (or inability) to improve or restore that patient's own physiologic mechanisms and resistance. Remember, for antibiotics to be effective, host resistance must be active no matter how good or how specific the medical treatments become. Osteopathic manipulative treatment enhances the homeostasis mechanisms of the patient who has the illness or dysfunction.

REFERENCES:

1. Owens C An Endocrine Interpretation of Chapman's Reflexes. Carmel CA, 1963.
2. Miller AJ: The lymphatic system and cardiac disease, in Lymph and the Lymphatic System, CC Thomas, 1968, pp 213-229.
3. Threefoot S: Lymphaticovenous communications, in Mayerson HS (ed) Lymph and the Lymphatic System. Springfield IL, CC Thomas, 1968, ch 2, pp 17-52.
4. Travell JG, Simons DG Myofascial Pain and Dysfunction: A Trigger Point Manual, Baltimore, Williams & Wilkins, 1983, p 672.
5. Barral JP, Mercier P Visceral Manipulation. Seattle WA, Eastland Press, 1988.
6. Herrmann E, The D.O., Oct. 1965, pp 163-4.

SYMPATHETIC INNERVATION OF THE GI TRACT AND PLAN FOR USE OF OSTEOPATHIC MANIPULATIVE TREATMENT

Anatomical Names	Anatomical No.	Group	Functional Innervation	Collateral Sympathetic Ganglion
Greater Splanchnic Nerve	T5-9	T5-9 (10)	Stomach, Liver Pancreas, Duodenum	Celiac Ganglion
Lesser Splanchnic Nerve	T10-11	T10-11 (12)	Small Intestines and Right Colon	Superior Mesenteric Ganglion
Least Splanchnic Nerve	T12	T12-L2	Left Colon and Pelvic Organs	Inferior Mesenteric Ganglion
Lumbar Splanchnic Nerve	L1-2			

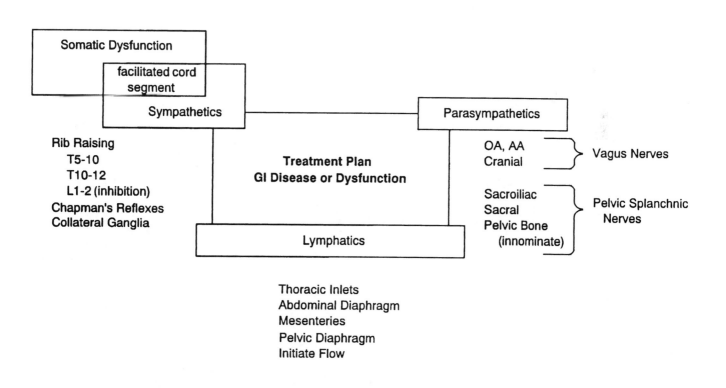

Somatic Dysfunction

facilitated cord segment

Sympathetics — Parasympathetics

Rib Raising
  T5-10
  T10-12
  L1-2 (inhibition)
Chapman's Reflexes
Collateral Ganglia

**Treatment Plan
GI Disease or Dysfunction**

OA, AA
Cranial — Vagus Nerves

Sacroiliac
Sacral
Pelvic Bone
(innominate) — Pelvic Splanchnic Nerves

Lymphatics

Thoracic Inlets
Abdominal Diaphragm
Mesenteries
Pelvic Diaphragm
Initiate Flow

NOTES:

OSTEOPATHIC CONSIDERATIONS
IN IRRITABLE BOWEL SYNDROME

"The high incidence of co-existing musculoskeletal defects as contributing factors makes this (irritable bowel) syndrome particularly interesting to the osteopathic physician."[1]

I. INTRODUCTION

The gastrointestinal tract is in a constant state of physiologic and biochemical activity, yet man is usually unaware of its function until it "rebels" causing gas, pain, or a change in frequency or type of bowel movements. It has been reported physicians will fail to discover an objective diagnosis or organic cause for 50% of people presenting with intestinal complaints.

For almost 100 years, osteopathic physicians have clinically used viscerosomatic reflexes to help them in their diagnosis and treatment of visceral and systemic disorders and disease. Through the work of Denslow, Hix, Korr, Patterson and Sato, these reflexes have been scientifically established. In spite of this evidence, these functional reflexes are seldom considered in present day medical texts and journals. They are also seldom referred to as an explanation for the pathogenesis of gastrointestinal disease processes, its symptoms or functional disorders.

In medical circles, "functional" often means that the symptoms can't be explained by present structural or biochemical knowledge; some physicians equate "functional" with psychological. One definition was found which conceded that there is a physiologic basis for the symptoms experienced by patients with functional disease.

Irritable bowel syndrome (IBS) is one of these functional diseases and has quite a common occurrence. It is a complex that is chronic, recurrent, intermittent, non-contagious and apparently non-pathological. Its importance to physicians is related to the fact that these patients present with symptoms which could be a part of any number of serious diseases. Major symptoms include complaints of abdominal pain usually related to meals and abnormal or irregular bowel habits, diarrhea and/or constipation. Secondary complaints may be distention of the abdomen, bloating, flatulence, and a sense of incomplete emptying of the bowel.

Once these symptoms are established in a person with IBS they rarely disappear; neither do they progress. If the symptoms of a person with IBS change radically, the physician must consider that a pathologic organic disease may be developing. These patients often have a high degree of stress in their lives.

They typically are rigid thinkers, orderly, and conscientious. They are usually preoccupied with planning and details. It has been reported that 70-80% of the patients with IBS have neurotic personalities but these traits are usually mild. Some studies have reported that psychiatric illness of the patient often precedes the diagnosis of irritable bowel syndrome. Actually many general practice physicians feel this psychiatric factor has been over-emphasized. Depression is common but it is often hidden by somatic complaints.

IBS should not be a wastebasket diagnosis given to a patient when symptoms do not fit other GI diseases. The typical patient with IBS is less than forty years of age but not over fifty, with recurrent abdominal pains and a history of an altered bowel habit. Since this history also fits so many organic pathologic diseases, the diagnosis of IBS is dependent upon the exclusion of pathologic problems. These organic disease possibilities include: Crohn's disease, ulcerative colitis, cancer of the colon, gastric/duodenal ulcer, cholelithiasis and amebiasis.

Unlike the diseases mentioned above, patients with the functional irritable bowel syndrome:

o .. Do not lose weight.
o .. Do not have fever.
o .. Do not have rectal ulcerations.
o .. Do not have rectal bleeding.
o .. Do not have anemia.
o .. Are not more likely to develop cancer of the colon than people who do not
      have IBS.

Early work-up of the patient relieves the anxiety of both the physician and the patient. It certainly prevents the physician from later performing piece-meal and repeated investigations because of an ambiguous understanding of the patient's symptoms and the chronic and frustrating nature of this "disease". Minimal basic work-up might include any or all of the following:

o .. CBC and Sed Rate--evidence of anemia or infection,
o .. Three stool specimens for occult blood, ova and parasites (including
      Giardia),
o .. Sigmoidoscopy and a warm slide prep for amoeba; biopsy if needed.
o .. A double contrast barium study looking for ulcerations, polyps, tumors or
      spasm.

If the patient also complains of dyspepsia, a gallbladder study should be ordered. If there is a complaint of diarrhea as well, a small bowel study should be ordered.

II. PHYSIOLOGY OF THE INTESTINAL TRACT

The intestines have both an extrinsic and an intrinsic control system. Intrinsically, the smooth muscle membranes of the bowel possess spontaneous electrophysiologic mechanisms capable of actively generating electrochemical gradients. These gradients can be stored and then discharged as electrical currents. The resultant cyclic activity of the smooth muscle of the gut is called "slow wave activity." Since spike potentials are produced in the same area of each slow wave and each results in a contraction, it is the slow wave frequency that determines the type of motor activity found in the intestines. There are two major slow wave frequencies: 6 and 3 cycle per minute. The normal smooth muscle membrane of the bowel in a person without bowel dysfunction or disease, has a balance of 90% of the 6 cpm and 10% of the 3 cpm slow waves. (See table page 113)

Functionally, these are the contractions normally found in the bowel:

o .. **"propulsive contractions"**--moves material through the gut.
o .. **"retropulsive contractions"**--moves contents back toward the stomach. The retropulsive contractions are more common in the ascending and transverse colon in order to slow the forward flow of the feces and to allow time for storage and additional time for absorption of fluids.
o .. **"non-propulsive contractions"**--just mix the contents of the bowel and move the material from one haustra to the next.
o .. **"mass movement"**--normally occur once or twice a day. This contraction squeezes off the main fecal mass stored in the cecum and ascending colon and moves it rapidly (in just a few minutes) over to the sigmoid colon.
o .. **"gastrocolic reflex"**--is a mass movement that occurs shortly after a meal. Unless it is frequent and excessive, it is considered a normal event. It is usually initiated by the hormone called gastrin.

The nervous control of the intestinal tract may be generally divided into two divisions, the intrinsic and the extrinsic portions. The function of the plexi, their nerve pathways and the overall benefit to the function of the entire body determines whether a given stress for a patient becomes conscious or remains subconscious; whether the reaction will be long-lasting or fleeting; or whether the response will set the stage for visceral pathology or not.

THE INTRINSIC NERVE CONTROL SYSTEM OF THE INTESTINES:

The intrinsic control system consists of the autonomic plexi within the wall of the intestines at which synapses between visceral afferents, the parasympathetic, and sympathetic nerve endings take place. At any one place along the intestine, the area's plexus modifies autonomic activity according to the local needs of that region of intestine. Smooth muscle in a section of the intestine can therefore respond to its local environment and can digest and move food along even if the extrinsic nerve supply has been surgically severed. Because this type of control is entirely unrelated to the external environment, it is termed vegetative and primitive. It is unrelated to the needs of the rest of the body as a whole.

THE EXTRINSIC NERVE CONTROL SYSTEM OF THE INTESTINES:

The GI tract coordinates its activity with other body systems and the external environment by way of the extrinsic autonomic nervous system. This extrinsic control of the intestine with its parasympathetic and sympathetic connections between the gut, the spinal cord, and the brain provides continuity and coordination between the internal control system and the rest of the body systems and the environment.

Because of its extrinsic connections, the GI tract can respond and its functions can be altered whenever the body is stressed psychologically, physically, chemically or traumatically.

THE SYMPATHETIC INNERVATION OF THE INTESTINES:

Sympathetic innervation to the GI tract has its origin in cord segments T5-L2 and innervates the intestines by way of the collateral sympathetic ganglia in the abdomen. The collateral ganglia are labeled celiac, superior mesenteric, and inferior mesenteric.

THE PARASYMPATHETIC INNERVATION OF THE INTESTINES:

Parasympathetic innervation is supplied by the vagus (cranial nerve X) to the upper GI, small intestines and right half of the colon; the pelvic splanchnic nerves (S2,3,4) supply parasympathetic innervation to the left half of the colon and the pelvis.

Research models indicate that dysfunction of the musculoskeletal system can produce visceral dysfunction in related viscera. This occurs via a somatovisceral reflex. If the musculoskeletal somatic dysfunction was removed "soon enough," the secondary visceral dysfunction disappeared.

If, however, the somatic dysfunction was left "too long," the visceral dysfunctions initially improved slightly but then become fully established again, even though the joint somatic dysfunction did not return. Apparently the reflex pattern was "burned into the nervous system" (learned). It has therefore been theorized that a directed program to keep people free from musculoskeletal somatic dysfunction could become a program for prevention of later internal disease. Further research is warranted in this area.

III. CHARACTERISTICS OF A PATIENT WITH IRRITABLE BOWEL SYNDROME:

The slow wave ratio in the intestine changes: In irritable bowel disease the patient's intestines have a different ratio of the 2 slow wave types: The 6 cpm waves are reduced from 90 to 60% and the 3 cpm waves are increased from 10 to 40%.

SLOW WAVES	NORMAL BOWEL PATIENT	IBS PATIENT
6 cpm	90%	60%
3 cpm	10%	40%

This new ratio hinders the forward flow of fecal contents and therefore produces a "functional obstruction." The change in the ratio of slow waves is present whether or not the patient is having symptoms. It is interesting to note that the increase in 3 cpm slow waves found in IBS patients is not found in patients with "pathologic diseases" such as ulcerative colitis or pancreatitis.

Patients with irritable bowel have the following functional characteristics:

Delayed and prolonged reactions to stimuli: In the fasting state, the spike potentials of a normal patient and the patient with irritable bowel syndrome are about the same. After a meal the normal patient has a rapid increase in spike potentials reaching a peak at about 40 minutes and shortly after returning to a normal resting level. This is considered a normal gastrocolic reflex. In the patient with irritable bowel syndrome, there is a delay and then a steady rise of the spike potentials. They only reach about 60% of their peak levels at 40 minutes and do not reach their peak until 90 minutes. The IBS patient's response is delayed and prolonged to normal changes in the internal environment. This is not in the best interest of the patient's total health.

Decreased nerve threshold levels encouraging excessive reaction to stimuli that would otherwise be considered to be normal: In a study demonstrating this phenomenon, a balloon was placed in the rectosigmoid region of normal patients and also in patients with IBS. Just placement of the balloon into that region of the intestine caused immediate and delayed contractions in the patient with irritable bowel syndrome. Then, with 60 cc of air in the balloon, 55% of the patients with IBS complained of pain while only 6% of the "normal patients" had pain. Even with only 20 cc of air in the balloon, 50% of the patients with IBS still had pain.

Apparently, excessive contractility of the bowel over a long period of time reduces the bowel's threshold to distension. As a result, even the usual amounts of intestinal gas cause the patient to have pain. The gut will remain overactive long after the stimulus is removed.

Intense emotional reactions: One of the most important factors determining "intensity of reaction" in patients with IBS, is the emotional level at which they live their lives. Anxiety should trigger sympathetic over activity and therefore reduced bowel function and activity should be expected.[2] Gillhorn at the University of Minnesota suggested that "the hypothalamus can tune against itself."[3] By this he meant that once the initial panic has subsided, the sympathetic effect is overruled by excessive induction of parasympathetic stimuli. A hypothalamic tuning can be either parasympathetic or sympathetic in response and may extend to related viscera such as the small intestine or the urinary tract.

Abnormal contraction patterns of the intestines: IBS patients may have "narrowing" of the intestines which produces diarrhea. This pattern is often found in the terminal small bowel and abnormal contractions in the cecum and ascending colon. They may have "segmentation" which is another abnormal pattern of contractions associated with the pain and flatulence of spastic constipation. This latter type of contraction causes "functional obstruction." If narrowing and segmentation occur together, the result is abdominal pain with constipation and stool with excessive mucus--but no blood.

Excessive gas: Man normally produces 6-8 liters of gas in the intestine every day, so gas is not abnormal in the intestinal tract.

The gas may be obtained from our external environment through swallowing air. This accounts mainly for the presence of nitrogen and oxygen. The gas produced in the normal bowel itself is the source of its carbon dioxide and hydrogen gas, but 30% of patients also produce methane gas. This gas is apparently produced through the action of some intestinal bacteria that still remain unidentified. If it were possible to develop a practical way to identify the people who produce methane gas, they could be watched closely; because 85% of these patients will develop cancer of the colon. People who develop cancer of the colon also produce methane gas in their colons.

All of the gases mentioned up to this point are odorless. Offensive odors from intestinal gas indicates the presence of trace gases which contain sulfa or various amine compounds and are more likely to be present when there is some bowel dysfunction.

Gas in the bowel can be absorbed if the partial pressures between the intestine and the gas in the capillary is appropriate, if the blood flow around the lumen is sufficient, and if the peristaltic activity is normal. Intestinal gas can be absorbed, passed rectally, belched, or, in certain cases, excreted by the lungs.

A medical researcher has observed and reported that patients with excessive flatulence often have increased low back lordosis. He might be describing the somatic effects of viscerosomatic reflexes activated through visceral afferent nerves from the colon and small intestine to the somatic nerves in the thoracolumbar area. The lordosis of the low back area might also be affecting the function of the intestine via a somatovisceral reflex.

Pain in the abdomen: Abdominal pain is a common complaint and results from a complex interplay of emotions, sensory factors and motor activity as well as neurologic and hormonal influences. 65% of the patients complain of pain below the umbilicus, 10% above the umbilicus: 25% complain of pain above and below the umbilicus at the same time.

The pain lasts for minutes in 30%, hours in 50% and days in 20%. Though pain located in the upper right quadrant does not occur very often, it must be carefully distinguished from pain caused by gallbladder disease or cholelithiasis. If a gallbladder is removed unnecessarily in a patient with IBS, the so-called "gallbladder pain" will increase because there is an increase, and constant release, of cholecystokinin (CCK) into the intestine after cholecystectomy. This enzyme increases bowel spasms.

Abdominal pain is due to various mechanisms:

Distention pain

Distention pain is not produced by stretching in the bowel wall, but by an attempt to stretch the mesenteries and serosal covering of the bowel beyond its normal length. Mesenteric and serosal tissues do not stretch. Distention is therefore limited by the serosal and mesenteric circumference allowed by the intestine. Lymphatic edema or venous congestion of the mesenteric tissue of the gut wall would reduce the amount of gas tolerated before pain from mesenteric pull would occur.

Contraction pain

Contraction pain is produced by contraction of the intestine on a fixed and incompressible mass of stool.

Compression pain

Compression pain is due to bowel contraction on an empty lumen and is apparently produced by pressure on sensitive mucosal and submucosal structures.

Both contraction pain and compression pain can be helped with the use of bulk and by reducing parasympathetic influence through some physical or medical means such as an anticholinergic agent.

IV. TREATMENT CONSIDERATIONS

Treatment of irritable bowel syndrome is important and often consists of some combination of OMT, dietary counselling, and medical prescription. The basic aim of all treatment is to remove the cause when a cause is present. When a cause is not evident, the treatment is symptomatic.

PHARMACOLOGIC TREATMENT :

o .. Antispasmodics taken before meals reduce the degree of gastrocolic reflex reaction in some people and also reduce the intralumenal pressure of the intestine.
o .. Tranquilizers or a tricyclic, like Elavil, may be helpful to control depression. Tranquilizers probably work best in right-sided abdominal pains because nervous, anxious patients usually have increased ileal intestinal flow. Many people think it is the atropine effect of these drugs that provide the beneficial effects on the GI tract.
o .. Antacids and/or H_2 inhibitors may be used to reduce the hydrogen radicals available for reaction with the bicarbonates found in the secretions of the gallbladder, pancreas and bowel. This reduces their reaction with bicarbonates to form water and carbon dioxide gas, further increasing intestinal gas and intestinal distention. Recall that antacids can themselves influence the bowel toward constipation or diarrhea depending on their formulation.

DIETARY TREATMENT:

o .. Non-absorbable bulk: Bulk in the diet in adequate amounts will provide 50% reduction in the bowel symptoms. Patients will complain of less abdominal pain because of reduced intralumenal pressure and they will have reduced mucorrhea.

o .. Wheat bran, 2 Tbls per day, divided and taken with meals, may be successful; or a polycarbophil tablet with meals may provide a gelatinous stool.

o .. Bulk should be started slowly and increased slowly because sudden increased bulk in the diet will itself upset the intestinal tract.

o .. Reduce the lactose intake. Lactose is the sugar found in milk. Lactase is a natural enzyme which permits normal breakdown of lactose. Lactase levels can be low in people anywhere in the world and is not an uncommon finding. The patient can be tested by removing milk from the diet for a 2-week period to see if the symptoms of bowel dysfunction are reduced. Lactase can also be added to milk and milk products to aid digestion.

o .. Restrict fat from the diet because fat stimulates bowel spasm and it also reacts with the bicarbonate radical in the small bowel to produce carbon dioxide gas.

OSTEOPATHIC MANIPULATIVE TREATMENT:

Irritable bowel syndrome is considered a "functional condition" without a known cause, but characterized by certain identifiable "functional and physiologic reactions." IBS patients react excessively to internal stimuli and are influenced heavily by external stimuli through the extrinsic autonomic control connections.

For these reasons, osteopathic manipulation is effective by improving function-structure relationships. Medicine, dietary modifications and osteopathic manipulative treatment in the management of this functional disease provide increased patient comfort and clinical improvement far beyond that expected by each type of treatment used alone. The physician's goals should be to normalize autonomic activity to the intestine, promote good lymphatic flow, and normalize joint somatic dysfunction--especially in the areas of sympathetic innervation to the GI tract. (See page 107) Treatment directed toward the support of the body's own self-regulatory mechanisms in a patient with a functional disease, is a practical conclusion based on an understanding of anatomy and physiology. Successful treatment of the patient with IBS often depends upon how much effort the physician exerts toward understanding the mechanisms of the disease process or the dysfunction. Osteopathic considerations in systemic dysfunction therefore should begin with a thorough understanding of the pathophysiology of IBS.

Support provided by specific osteopathic manipulative techniques is designed to:

o .. balance the extrinsic autonomic nervous system, both sympathetic and parasympathetic.
o .. relieve lymphatic and venous congestion in the intestinal tract.
o .. remove chronic joint somatic dysfunctions which play a role in perpetuating detrimental facilitated cord segments.

MANIPULATION AFFECTING THE SOMATIC COMPONENT:

It has been reported that somatic dysfunction can be associated with, or potentiated by, visceral dysfunction; and a vicious cycle of viscerosomatic and somatovisceral reflexes can be postulated. Palpable somatic paraspinal findings produced by viscerosomatic reflex pathways can be used as clues to the location of internal visceral dysfunction. General stress, structural problems, abnormal posture, and trauma can each produce spinal joint somatic dysfunction. Somatic dysfunction of joints is also associated with the facilitated segment and sympathicotonia.

MANIPULATION AFFECTING SYMPATHETICS:

Though sympathetic activity may help in "fight or flight" situations, its perpetuation is detrimental to the healing process. With the understanding that hypersympathetic activity is present in all dysfunctions and diseases, hypersympathetic activity can be treated by osteopathic manipulation at a number of sites and in the following ways:

Rib raising and segmental osteopathic manipulative treatment:

In IBS, supine paraspinal "rib raising" inhibition (see page 195) and soft tissue to the thoracolumbar area (T10-L2) is especially beneficial.

Treatment of the collateral sympathetic ganglia:

Use inhibitory ventral abdominal techniques. In a patient with IBS, the midline area between the xiphoid process and the umbilicus is tense to palpation and it is tender to the patient even when palpated lightly. Just a few seconds of steady "humane" pressure over the ganglia reduces the palpable tension and relieves the patient's subjective discomfort.

<hr>

Treatment of Chapman's reflexes:

<hr>

Chapman's reflexes are believed to be produced by viscerosomatic, visceral afferent induced reflexes referred from visceral dysfunction to the soma. They can be very specifically mapped out on the body and charts are available. (Refer to pages 232 and 233.)

Most physicians use the anterior points to identify the organ which may have dysfunction. Anterior points for the small intestine refer to the anterior intercostal spaces 8, 9, and 10 on each side. Chapman's reflexes from the colon are found in the iliotibial bands, a 2-inch strip on the lateral side of each thigh. These can be treated with soft tissue kneading, a mechanical percussion hammer, or other types of vibration to produce an effective somatovisceral influence on the sympathetic innervation to the colon.

MANIPULATION AFFECTING PARASYMPATHETICS:

The effects of manipulation directed toward normalization of parasympathetic activity have relatively little experimental verification. Clinical effects, however, are observed. The pelvic splanchnic nerve provides parasympathetic innervation to the left half of the colon and pelvic organs while the vagus provides innervation to the rest of the GI tract.

<hr>

Treatment of somatic dysfunction of the sacroiliac joints:

<hr>

The pelvic splanchnics have an S2,3,4 origin while the sacroiliac joint incorporates sacral segments 1, 2, and 3. Because of this anatomic proximity, IBS symptomatology is considered to be affected by somatic dysfunctions of the sacrum--torsion, rotations, shears--or by sacroiliac somatic dysfunction-- anterior, posterior and superior innominate shear. Therefore, somatic dysfunctions of these areas are specifically manipulated to normalize the parasympathetic activity to the left colon.

Anterior pressure and rocking over the sacrum of a patient, prone on the table, has been found to clinically modify parasympathetic tone, even in the absence of specific sacral somatic dysfunction.

Treatment of the OA, AA, C2 and use of condylar decompression:

The right vagus nerve supplies parasympathetic innervation to the right half of the colon and small intestines and may be affected by somatic dysfunction at the OA, AA, C2 and the lambdoidal suture of the cranium, especially in the area of the jugular foramen and the occipitomastoid suture. Osteopathic manipulation of somatic dysfunction palpable in these areas is effective in normalizing parasympathetic activity to the proximal GI tract and the right half of the colon.

MANIPULATION AFFECTING THE LYMPHATIC SYSTEM:

With organ and tissue dysfunction there will be lymphatic and venous congestion. This interferes with blood, nerve, nutrition and oxygenation of tissues and results in the increase of toxic waste products in and around the cells. Congestion also hinders the plexi for intrinsic autonomic control and reduces the intestine's ability to inform the CNS of the exact nature of local conditions. This information is necessary so that the local responses will be appropriate to the needs of the entire body and to its external environment.

Techniques often used to affect the lymphaticovenous system include:

Soft tissue treatment to the thoracolumbar junction:

This prepares the fascias and other soft tissues for abdominal diaphragmatic redoming.

Treatment to the thoracic inlet and redoming of the abdominal diaphragm:

Basic for opening the pathway for lymphatic drainage and for support of the extrinsic lymphatic pump.

Ventral abdominal techniques:

These are directed toward the mesenteries to help relieve the congestive effects of visceroptosis, to free the fascial planes of the mesenteries, to reduce abdominal pain, to provide better circulation to the intestines, to improve lymphatic flow, and to insure more appropriate autonomic responses.

VI. SUMMARY

Osteopathic physicians have the ability to use proven pharmacologic and dietary treatment wisely and to provide manipulative support to the patient's own body mechanisms. The body also has inherent mechanisms to combat dysfunction or disease. They recognize that these mechanisms may not always be working at their optimal level of efficiency as evidenced by the wide variety and range of responses observed in a group of patients exposed to a similar stress. It is easy to comprehend that inherent compensatory mechanisms often require assistance to permit them to function at their optimal levels and capacities.

The result of osteopathic manipulative treatment is palpable in the tissues. Functional changes are clinically observable and subjective improvements are voiced by the patients. Good results are not limited to the office visit or the immediate post-treatment period, but continue on; apparently it is possible to tune the intrinsic mechanisms to a new level of performance.

Manipulation, as a part of the management of a patient with irritable bowel syndrome, allows the physician to better control that patient's responses to life-stress and helps to give the patient physiologic relief from his symptoms. Osteopathic manipulation benefits the patient by providing relaxation, normalizing extrinsic and intrinsic autonomic control mechanisms and relieving congestion.

Osteopathic manipulation is directed toward the patient, for the patient who has dysfunction or disease. It allows a personal manipulative prescription for the specific needs of that particular patient.

RECOMMENDED READING FOR OSTEOPATHIC CONSIDERATIONS IN PATIENTS WITH IRRITABLE BOWEL SYNDROME:

Sleisenger MH, Fordtran JS Gastrointestinal Diseases. Saunders Co, 3rd ed, 1983.

Sernka T, Jacobson E Gastrointestinal Physiology. Williams and Wilkins, 1983.

Battle WM, Kohen S, Snape W: Inhibition of postprandial colonic immobility after ingestion of an amino acid mixture. Digestive Diseases and Sciences Sep 1980; 25(9): 647-652.

Ritchie JA, Truelove SE: Comparisons of various treatment for irritable syndrome. British Medical Journal Nov 15, 1980; 281: 1317-1319.

Sullivan M, Kohen S, Snape W: Colonic myoelectric activity in irritable bowel syndrome. Effects of Eating and Anticholinergics: 878-883.

Kailbinger H, Weilkrauch TR: Drugs increasing gastrointestinal pharmacology. Karger, Basel 1982; 25: 61-72.

Patriquin D: Eponym syndrome blindness: Is there a cure? <u>JAOA</u> Mar 1984;
    83(7): 516/95-521-100.

Lazarus B: Overview of irritable bowel syndrome. <u>JAOA</u> 6/11-20/11.

Masterson E: Irritable bowel syndrome: An osteopathic approach. <u>Osteopathic
    Annals</u> Jan 1984; 12(1):˜12/21-18/31.

Denslow JS: Functional colitis: Etiology. <u>AAO Yearbook</u> Vol 1, 1965, pp
    192-197.

McBain: Treatment of functional colon. <u>AAO Yearbook</u> Vol 1, 1965, pp 190-
    191.

Round Table: Upper gastrointestinal diseases. <u>Clinical Challenges</u> 1984; 1(3):
    2-83.

Burnstock G, O'Brien R, Vrbova G: <u>Somatic and Autonomic Nerve-Muscle
    Interactions</u>. Amsterdam, Elsevier, 1983, pp 383-351.

REFERENCES:

1. Strong WB: Disorders of the digestive system, in Hoag JM (ed)
        <u>Osteopathic Medicine</u>. New York, McGraw-Hill, 1969, ch 38, p 595.

2. Almy TP et al: Alternatives In Colon Function. <u>Gastroenterology</u> 1949;
        12: 425-436.

3. Gilhorn in <u>Autonomic Imbalance In The Hypothalamus</u>. U of Minnesota
        Press, 1957.

OSTEOPATHIC CONSIDERATIONS
IN GENITOURINARY TRACT DISORDERS

"The more the osteopathic urologist makes use of manipulative therapy, the sooner (s)he becomes aware that special manipulative measures can improve and sometimes effect recovery from various genitourinary disorders."[1]

I. INTRODUCTION

Poor posture and compromised body mechanics have long been implicated in a wide range of functional disorders including those affecting the genitourinary system. Goldthwait in the text, <u>Essentials of Body Mechanics in Health and Disease</u>, discusses the role of bad body mechanics, chronic passive congestion, the failure of the diaphragmatic pump and pressure on sympathetic ganglia as factors promoting irregularities in organ function. "These disturbances, if continued long enough, may lead to diseases in later life. Faulty body mechanics in early life, then, becomes a vital factor in the production of the vicious cycle of chronic disease and presents the chief point of attack in its prevention."[2]

Specifically, Goldthwait suggests that one of the first goals of treatment might be to restore good body mechanics:

> "A loose kidney is found almost always with a faulty posture.   The drooped thorax obliterates the forward thrust of the ribs and relaxes the diaphragm, thus pushing the liver downward on the kidney to the right. Because of this pressure, the protecting fat is rapidly lost and ptosis of the kidney follows. Chronic passive congestion, kinked ureters, hydronephrosis, orthostatic albuminuria, urinary stasis, stones and infection are possible outcomes, since function of the kidneys is dependent on full blood and nerve supply and on free drainage--all of which ptosis may disturb. The normal position of the kidneys can be restored, and the protecting fat replaced, by relieving the downward pressure of bad body mechanics."[3]

Osteopathic considerations therefore include not only a complete history and examination of genitourinary (GU) structures and/or functions, but also extend to the posture of the patient and to related somatic dysfunction (neural, lymphatic, and circulatory elements) involved in homeostasis of these organs. The importance of the thoracic and pelvic diaphragms and the fascias surrounding the GU organs is crucial to a treatment protocol stressing homeostatic support of the patient with GU dysfunction.

This section delineates general somatic, autonomic, circulatory, and fascial considerations as they pertain to the pathophysiology occurring in patients with genitourinary disorders.

II. KIDNEYS, URETERS AND BLADDER (KUB)

The kidneys control both volume and composition of body fluids by regulating the excretion of water and solutes. Urine, formed in the kidneys, contains metabolic waste products, foreign substances (including pharmacologic by-products) and other water-soluble constituents of the body in quantities depending upon homeostatic needs and the functional ability of the kidney at any given time. The kidneys are also involved in blood pressure control and red blood cell production.

The kidneys are retroperitoneal structures encased in fatty tissue. A tough areolar fascia surrounds the kidney, splits into two layers which are not continuous inferiorly, allowing the kidneys to move downward with the diaphragm during inhalation. This factor is utilized in the routine physical examination by having the patient take a deep inhalation so the kidney will move downward and allow itself to be more easily palpated. A "floating kidney" may be detected in this manner and kidney enlargement may reflect hydronephrosis, cancer, or polycystic kidney disease. Because of the continuity of fascias, diaphragmatic descent is the chief factor in venous as well as lymphatic return from the GU viscera. Diaphragmatic motion can be reduced by somatic dysfunction of the thoracolumbar junction or lower ribs, hyperlordosis, somatic dysfunction affecting the phrenic nerve (C3-5) and/or spasm of the quadratus lumborum or psoas muscles.

The psoas muscle courses obliquely causing lateral displacement of the lower poles of each kidney. Any limitation of motion in the upper lumbar vertebrae (as can occur with psoas spasm) will result in fascial restriction of the motion of the kidneys. The ureters adhere directly to the peritoneum and descend on the psoas fascia, cross the genitofemoral nerve, and continue into the pelvis to the bladder. Psoas contracture or spasm may also cause the fascias to adversely affect ureteral function.

The bladder and urethra carry with them the same innervation as the systems from which they were embryologically derived. The sphincter, trigone and ureteral orifices are activated by the sympathetics (whose cell bodies originate from cord segments T12-L2) and are inhibited by the parasympathetics (originating from S2-4). The bladder wall is activated by the parasympathetics and inhibited by the sympathetics.

SYMPATHETICS:

Sympathetic innervation to the kidneys and ureters begins in sympathetic cell bodies in the spinal cord at the level of T10-L1. The preganglionic fibers for kidney and upper ureter synapse primarily in the superior mesenteric collateral ganglion; while those for the lower ureter synapse primarily in the inferior mesenteric ganglion. The sympathetic preganglionic fibers to the bladder arise from cell bodies in the T12-L2 level of the cord and synapse in the inferior mesenteric collateral ganglion. Sympathetic stimulation causes vasoconstriction of afferent arterioles, decreases the glomerular filtration rate (GFR), and results in decreased urine volume.[4] This response is exaggerated with emotional stress.[5] Increased sympathetic tone decreases ureteral peristaltic waves and may cause ureterospasm. Ureteral stimulation, as might occur with a ureteral stone, selects the kidney as a target organ for sympathetic discharge triggered by rostral reflex centers.[6] Functional urinary obstruction can occur with visceromotor reflex alterations arising from somatic dysfunction.[7,8,9] It also relaxes the bladder wall, which may result in reflux and incomplete emptying of the bladder. Guyton suggests a role for chronic sympathicotonia to the kidneys in the etiology of essential hypertension. His physiology text suggests that essential hypertension is probably invoked by a "*functional retention*" of water and salt by the kidneys:

". . . experiments show when sympathetic nerves to kidneys are stimulated continuously for several weeks, renal retention of fluid occurs and causes chronically elevated arterial pressure as long as the sympathetic stimulation continues. Therefore, it is possible for nervous stimulation of the kidneys to cause chronic elevation of arterial pressure."[10]

Anterior Chapman's viscerosomatic reflexes[11] for the bladder are located periumbilically with those referable to the kidney located on the ipsilateral side, one inch lateral and one inch superior to the umbilicus.

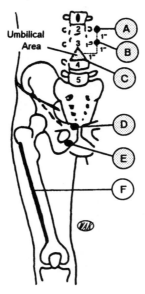

CHAPMAN'S POINTS RELATED TO THE GENITO-URINARY SYSTEM (T10-L2; Superior Mesenteric Ganglion, Inferior Mesenteric Ganglion)

Key to palpating pertinent points:

A. Adrenals
B. Kidneys
C. Bladder
D. Prostate or Broad Ligament
E. Gonads
F. Uterus

Posterior Chapman's points are located in the intertransverse space (midway between spines and transverse process tips of L1-2 and T12-L1 respectively.

PARASYMPATHETICS:

The parasympathetics which supply the kidney arise from the vagus nerve. The proximal portion of the ureters are supplied by the vagus and the distal portion by the pelvic splanchnic nerves (S2-4). The bladder's parasympathetic nerves come only from the pelvic splanchnic nerves. It is not known how the parasympathetic nerves affect the kidney but in the ureters they maintain normal peristaltic waves.

As the bladder fills, visceral afferents in the bladder wall transmit impulses to L1-2 to sense "fullness"; at the same time, visceral afferents to S2-4 initiate a parasympathetic reflex to increase the bladder wall tone and, eventually, a simultaneous relaxation of the internal urethral sphincter. Then, with the voluntary relaxation of the external urethral sphincter via impulses from S2-4 (the pudendal nerve) and the simultaneous sympathetic relaxation to the external urinary sphincter, micturation takes place.[12] While the external urethral sphincter is primarily under voluntary control, sympathetic relaxation must also simultaneously occur during voiding.

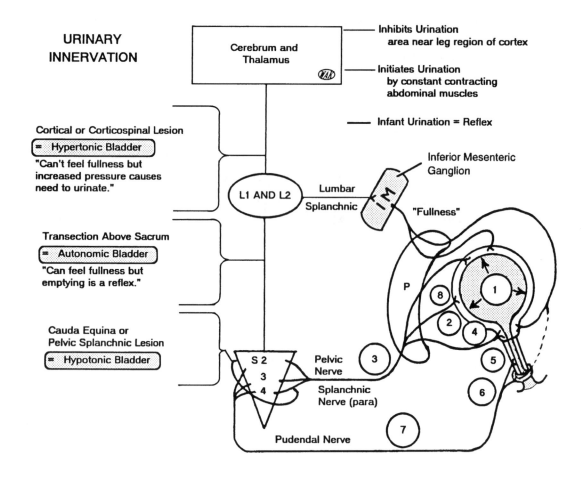

126

LYMPHATICS:

Renal lymphatics draining the capsule and parenchyma flow into the preaortic nodes before travelling up the thoracic duct to the subclavian vein. The synchronous motion of thoracic and pelvic diaphragms is vital to lymphatic drainage from the urinary system. The purpose of the lymphatics is to drain the capsule and parenchyma, acting as a "safety valve system that aids in the clearance of waste products of the kidney as well as fluid, electrolytes, and infectious or antibiotic products." It has been shown that during acute ureteral obstruction, renal hilar lymph flow increases up to 300%.[13] With renal vein or ureteral obstruction, capsular lymphatics are known to dilate to prevent renal damage while Babics and Renyl-Vamos ascribe the survival and continued performance of the hydronephrotic kidney to the fact that "urine passes from the renal pelvis into the interstitial space of the kidney where it is continuously absorbed into the lymphatics."

The countercurrent exchange concept of urine formation visualizes the vasa recta as important in carrying off salt and water. An osmotic gradient must be maintained between the interstitium and the plasma for these vessels to function properly. This gradient is maintained only through adequate lymphatic drainage. Interference with lymphatic drainage has been shown to cause a rise in the oncotic pressure of the interstitium and an inability of the kidney to concentrate urine.

VISCEROSENSORY/VISCEROMOTOR REFLEXES:

The renal visceromotor reflex will cause increased tonus to the thoracolumbar junction and a positive Lloyd's punch test. The renal viscerosensory reflex is usually described as an ache rather than as a pain. It may refer only to the thoracolumbar area, the flank, or both. The ureteral viscerosensory reflex (ureterocolic) usually extends from the lumbar region and the iliac fossa over the front of the abdomen and into the scrotum or labia. The ureteromotor reflex also causes the abdominal, erector spinae and the cremasteric muscles to become tense. As a stone passes through the ureters, palpatory changes from visceromotor reflexes will progress from T10 into the lumbar region.

SOMATIC SYSTEM:

External sphincter tone relies on reasonable innervation from the pudendal nerve (S2-4). When there is a sudden increase in intra-abdominal pressure, the pelvic diaphragm with the external sphincters will contract in response to a protective reflex arc. If the contraction of the sphincter is inadequate, urinary incontinence may occur when that person coughs, sneezes or lifts a heavy object. This problem is more frequent in female patients.

127

When the pelvic diaphragm has increased tone or is spastic and can not work synchronously with the thoracic diaphragm, there will often be a resultant elevation of intra-abdominal/intrapelvic pressure. This can aggravate the symptoms in patients with inguinal or esophageal hernias. Pelvic floor tension myalgia can also lead to a variety of urinary symptoms ranging from testicular ache to frequency and urgency.[14]

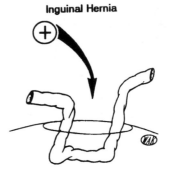

Inguinal Hernia

Treatment Protocol

1. Reduce Hernia
2. Remove Stresses on Pelvic Floor
3. Diminish Intra-abdominal Pressure
4. Elective Surgical Repair

Postural disorders, particularly short leg syndrome, and psoas spasm frequently cause backache and when accompanied by functionally induced urinary changes are often misconstrued as urinary tract infection.[15]

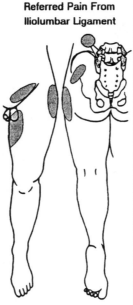

Referred Pain From Iliolumbar Ligament

The iliolumbar ligament is one of the earliest structures strained in postural decompensation and should be palpated in all patients in which this is suspected. Pain may be localized to the sites of attachment or may refer into the lateral thigh and/or groin. X rays may show ligament calcification or bony exostosis in cases of chronic postural strain. Treatment of acute symptomatology may include counterstrain, NSAIDs and occasionally local injection. However, the underlying postural cause should be identified and treated. Appropriate orthotic adjuncts--heel lift in patient with short leg syndrome or a Levitor® in patient with hyperlordosis or spondylolisthesis-- is often necessary to prevent reoccurances.

Pain pattern modified from George S. Hackett MD, FACS

Postural disorders have further been implicated as a cause of pelvic diaphragm tension myalgia, whose symptoms are frequently misdiagnosed as prostatitis.[16]

Iliolumbar ligament strain is also a frequent consequence of postural disorders and is acutely activated by lifting. Because of the mechanism of onset and of the referred pain pattern into the groin region, iliolumbar ligament strain is often perceived by the patient to be caused by an inguinal hernia.

Somatic dysfunction of the pubic symphysis with tension in the urogenital diaphragm or the puboprostatic or pubovesicular ligaments may cause dysuria, urgency or frequency of urination. This may be experienced by postpartum women or patients who have had either cystoscopy or perineal surgery wherein the somatic dysfunction can be obtained while they are being incorrectly helped out of the stirrups following the procedure. In children, this somatic dysfunction has been associated with nocturnal enuresis.

Trigger points in the lower abdomen[17] may cause urinary frequency and urgency, sphincter spasm, and residual urine, or pain in the urinary bladder. In one reported case, treatment of a trigger point in an old appendectomy scar relieved the symptoms of frequency and urgency and increased the patient's bladder capacity by 45%.[18]

III. THE GENITAL/REPRODUCTIVE SYSTEM

The Mullerian and Wolffian ducts are of epiblastic origin so the muscles that surround these ducts in the pelvis are innervated by the dermal systems distribution of sympathetic nerves. The Mullerian ducts become the fallopian tubes and form the uterus and vagina. The Wolffian duct gives origin to the vas deferens and ejaculatory duct.

SYMPATHETICS AND PARASYMPATHETICS:

The fallopian tubes, uterus, vagina, vas deferens and seminal vesicles (with the exception of the cervix) are activated by sympathetics having cell body origins from T11 to T12 in the spinal cord. Because of their embryologic origin, the sympathetic nerves are the only innervation to most of these structures; however, the cervix, vagina, clitoris and walls of the urethra are supplied with a few parasympathetic fibers from S2-4. The majority of the synapses between pre- and post-ganglionic sympathetic fibers occur in the inferior mesenteric ganglion. A separate nerve supply for the cervix is created by the pelvic splanchnic nerves (parasympathetic) and activates the cervix while producing some inhibitory influence on the body of the uterus.

The prostate, as well as the Cowper and Bartholin glands, have secretory sympathetic fibers originating from T12-L2. Stimulation of the hypogastric plexus of nerves, which carries the sympathetic fibers from T12-L2, produces true glandular secretion from the prostate gland structure while stimulation of the pudendal nerve forces the secretions out the urethra by contracting musculature.

Anterior Chapman's points to the prostate or broad ligament are located in the myofascial tissues along the posterior margin of the iliotibial band. Tenderness to moderate pressure over this area or tenderness and a palpatory sense of resistance to palpation over the inferior mesenteric collateral ganglion or the T12-L2 paraspinal tissues should increase the level of suspicion of dysfunction arising from one of these structures.

Stimulation of parasympathetic fibers from S2-4 will relax the smooth musculature of the corpora cavernosa in the penis and results in an erection as the muscle fills with blood. The penis also has sympathetic fibers from L1-2 which innervate the smooth musculature involved in orgasm and ejaculation. Impotence may be associated with reduction of parasympathetic tone resulting in the impairment of erectile capabilities; or it may be associated with reduction of sympathetic activity (as occurs in diabetics), resulting in dysfunctional ejaculation disorders. Hypersympathetic tone producing premature ejaculation could easily come from facilitation of segments at the thoracolumbar level, especially L1-2.

The testes and ovaries (gonadal tissues) produce hormonal secretions which have a marked influence on the growth and energies of the individual. These secretions are under the control of the sympathetic fibers, originating in the T10-11 spinal cord area. They synapse in the superior mesenteric collateral ganglion. These nerves produce their effect primarily through their action on the gonadal vascular supply. Anterior Chapman's points associated with the gonadal tissues are located on the superior surface of the pubic bones. Parasympathetic supply is from S2-4 but its effects are unknown except for the fact that it does not affect secretory activity of the gonads.

LYMPHATICS:

Pelvic organs are dependent upon the synchronous motion of the active thoracic diaphragm with the passive pelvic diaphragm during respiration. The prostate actually fills an anatomical urogenital defect in the pelvic diaphragm and is continuously massaged by the passive motion imparted by respiratory activity when the pelvic floor is free to move.

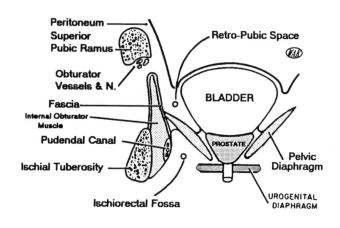

This anatomical and functional symbiosis is considered necessary for the establishment of effective lymphatic flow.

130

Pelvic congestion also plays a major role in the symptomatology noted in patients with dysmenorrhea, ovarian cysts, or with premenstrual syndrome. Increased vaginal leukorrhea has been associated with the venous and lymphatic stasis of pelvic congestion.[19] In premenstrual syndrome (PMS) congestion and fluid retention are responsible for generalized edema, backache, headache, mastalgia, pelvic pain, nervousness, irritability, emotional instability, depression and weight gain. The syndrome has a postulated hormonal basis, but hormonal manipulation has been less helpful in the treatment than would be expected from this theoretical etiology. The adjunctive use of diuretics at the first indication of PMS and the use of NSAIDs has also been beneficial in some cases through their effects in modifying congestion, inflammation and prostaglandin activity.

VISCEROSENSORY AND VISCEROMOTOR:

Viscerosensory reflexes from the gonads are of considerable clinical importance. They produce pain in the groin which at times seems to radiate down the thigh. The etiology of pain referred from the iliolumbar ligaments should be carefully considered in the differential diagnosis of genitourinary tract disorders. Visceromotor reflexes from the genitourinary tract cause rigidity in the lowest portion of the abdominal musculature and in the T10-11 paraspinal musculature.

Motor reflexes from the uterus are not very pronounced, however the sensory reflex is definite and well recognized; pain is a common sign in both uterine and tubal disorders. Pain arising from the fallopian tubes may be felt in the flank, iliac fossa, and down the anterior thigh to the knee. Uterine pain is felt in the thoracolumbar junction, the abdomen, and occasionally in the sacral region. Segmental referred pain[20] and spinal palpatory changes from the female reproductive tract has been most frequently described as being located at T10 for the ovaries, T11-12 for fallopian tubes, T10-L1 for the uterus, and S2-4 for the cervix.

The prostate displays viscerosensory reflexes, traveling via its sympathetic and parasympathetic routes, as pain in both the thoracolumbar and sacral regions. Pain may also be felt in the glans penis with accompanying urinary frequency and rectal discomfort because of the common connection of these tissues with the pelvic nerve.

"The penis is more often the subject of reflex sensation than the cause of it."[21] Because it is bound to urogenital and rectal structures by filaments of the pelvic nerve, it is subject to reflex sensory disturbances originating from dysfunction of renal, ureteral, bladder, urethral, testicular or prostatic tissues. Infection or inflammation of these structures will facilitate the L1-2 segments causing almost continuous sexual desire.

The mechanisms of many "aphrodisiacs" can be traced to their ability to irritate or inflame the bladder to set up this type of facilitation. The location of the inner thigh "erogenous zones" also correlates with areas which when stimulated would enhance neural input into the cord at these levels.

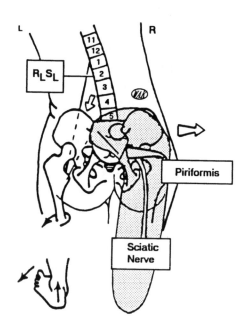

SOMATIC:

Dysfunction of the psoas muscle has been implicated in gynecologic dysfunction because of its anatomic proximity to affect various physiologic mechanisms important to this system - vascular, neurologic, and lymphatic. Chronic psoas spasm has been reported to cause anovulation[22] and is also reflective of the so called genitoiliopsoatic syndrome wherein chronic ovarian inflammation causes reflex psoas spasm.[23]

Postural disorders, myofascial trigger points and pelvic somatic dysfunction also contribute to pain patterns and symptoms commonly associated with genitoreproductive tract disorders. Short leg syndrome is not only implicated in low back and lower abdominal pain but also in pelvic pain.[24] Symptoms of dysmenorrhea are frequently intensified by trigger points in the lower rectus abdominus muscles.[25] Somatic dysfunction of the sacroiliac joint or muscle spasm in that area may refer pain suggestive of uterine cervical disorders.[26]

OTHER:

Psychoemotional factors play a very significant role in genitoreproductive functions. Reduction of stress has been a valuable therapeutic element in caring for patients with functional infertility, frigidity and impotence.

IV. TREATMENT CONSIDERATIONS

The specific techniques provided are much less important than accomplishing goals which support patient homeostasis and maximize structure/function relationships.

PLAN FOR OSTEOPATHIC MANIPULATION OF PATIENT WITH UROLOGICAL DYSFUNCTION:

```
                    C3-5  (Phrenic Nerve)
                    Sacroiliacs (Pudendal Nerve, S2,3,4)
```

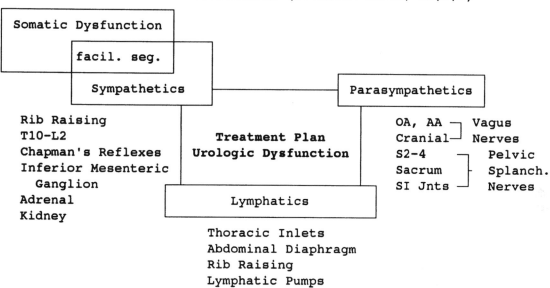

SYMPATHETIC (PATHO)PHYSIOLOGY:

↑ Tone:

    1. ↑ Afferent Arteriole Constriction to Kidney
    2. Ureterospasm and ↓ Peristalsis of Ureters
    3. Relaxation of Bladder Wall Leading to Reflux
    4. ↑ Tone to External Urinary Sphincter

Effects:

    ↓ GFR → ↓ Urinary Output
    Elevates Blood Pressure
    Ureterospasm → ↓ Urine Flow through the Ureters
    Encourages Incomplete Emptying of Bladder
    Encourages Ureteral/Prostatic Reflux from Bladder
    Complaints of Premature or Retrograde Ejaculation

LYMPHATIC (PATHO)PHYSIOLOGY:

Impaired Lymphatic Flow Effects:

1. ↑ Oncotic Interstitial Pressure →
   Disrupted Countercurrent Exchange →
   ↓ Ability to Concentrate Urine Properly
2. ↑ Risk of Kidney Damage Because of Ureteral
   Obstruction

PARASYMPATHETIC (PATHO)PHYSIOLOGY:

↑ Tone:

1. ↑ Peristalsis of Ureters
2. ↑ Bladder Wall Tone
3.   Relaxes Internal Urinary Sphincter

↓ Tone:

1.   Incomplete Emptying of Bladder
2.   Impotence
3.   Tightens Internal Urinary Sphincter

URINARY TRACT INFECTIONS (UTI):

Urinary tract infections (UTI) are among the most frequent bacterial infections encountered and the most common disease process occurring in the GU system. UTIs are ten times more frequent in women than men. If there is a kidney infection and/or posterior peritoneal irritation, the Lloyd's punch test will usually be positive. Chapman's reflexes, collateral ganglion involvement, and the pattern of segmental somatic dysfunction help establish a correct differential diagnosis and correlate with the extent of the inflammation. Except for some simple UTIs, investigation is necessary to detect obstructive uropathies, urinary calculi, or other predisposing or perpetuating factors; further investigation is also statistically warranted in male patients with UTI. It should be noted that chronic bacterial prostatitis is the most common cause of relapsing bladder infection (cystitis) in males.

Osteopathic considerations include ruling out pubic symphyseal and pelvic floor somatic dysfunctions which may produce symptoms of dysuria and frequency. Treatment of pelvic floor somatic dysfunction is helpful in reducing specific mechanical contributions to symptoms as well as aiding in the relief of the prostatic congestion that these somatic dysfunctions can produce.

Incomplete emptying, reflux and loss of normal ureteral peristalsis are risk factors for ascending infection and should be addressed by treatment to both the thoracolumbar junction (T10-L2) and the sacroiliac joint (S1-3). Treating a patient to reduce sympathetic hyperactivity is felt to help the body deal with local and systemic infections by removing a factor hindering tissue defense and promoting mechanisms which lead to reduced tissue congestion and adequate tissue antibiotic levels.

Modification of urinary pH is often an effective treatment of urinary tract infections and can be accomplished with medication or to a lesser degree, with cranberry juice. Intake of fluids in general is important.

RENAL DISEASE:

All appropriate measures to prevent or limit renal structural changes in infectious or obstructive uropathies should be taken and this goal is maximized with early recognition of GU dysfunctional states. With regard to acute glomerulonephritis, Osteopathic Medicine notes[27] that somatic dysfunction "at T11, T12, and L1 should be considered as an etiologic component in view of the proven pathologic changes apparently associated with such (somatic dysfunction). In this regard manipulative treatment might well be a preventive aid." A similar statement is made with regard to acute pyelonephritis, "Patients having (T11, T12, and L1 somatic dysfunction) are much more vulnerable to acute pyelonephritis and they are much less likely to respond to treatment, if spinal manipulation is not part of the program of management."[28] Even when significant structural change has occurred, as in chronic glomerulonephritis, OMT to these areas to limit dysfunctional reflex activity while "not curative ... will improve renal circulation and is considered decongestive."[29]

Renal failure with resultant azotemia and uremia is "one example in which applied osteopathic manipulative therapy has in the past produced dramatic results."[30] OMT to the T10-L2 region in an attempt to maximize renal circulation in patients with renal failure "permit a much faster convalescence."[31] Sterritt reports a case study in which OMT to the thoracolumbar area is credited with improving urinary output and substantially decreasing a critically elevated BUN.[32]

The general concept of the osteopathic manipulative approach is that by eliminating the somatic dysfunction component with its related effect on neural, lymphatic and vascular elements the diseased kidney will function maximally within its existing structural limitations. Beyond this, any failed or incomplete homeostatic mechanisms are replaced by artificial mechanisms - medication, correction of electrolyte imbalance and acidosis, and potentially dialysis. To this end, manipulative treatment to assist the homeostatic responses of patients with renal disorders is not disease-specific but rather host-specific.

135

PROSTATITIS:

Prostatitis is not one disease. Common prostatitis syndromes include acute bacterial prostatitis, chronic bacterial prostatitis, nonbacterial prostatitis, and prostatodynia.[33] Treatment varies depending on the type of syndrome present.

Acute bacterial prostatitis is characterized by fever, chills, myalgia and/or arthralgias, dribbling and/or slowed urinary stream, perineal and low back pain. It may be accompanied by gross hematuria. The gland will be tender, warm and swollen to palpation. Digital massage in an acutely infected gland should be avoided because of the risk of bacteremia. Because cystitis usually accompanies bacterial prostatitis, culture of voided bladder urine usually allows identification of the pathogen. The chemical structure of trimethoprim permits it to penetrate the prostatic wall achieving high levels in the prostatic secretions. This makes trimethoprim or the combination of trimethoprim with sulfamethoxazole the drugs of choice at the present time. OMT addressing the ischiorectal fossa, T12-L2 and S2-4 regions is the manipulative treatment of choice in maximizing prostatic levels of antibiotics and in assisting the body's natural defenses. Inadequate prostatic treatment in these patients can lead to chronic relapsing urinary tract infections from ascending infection.

Many patients with chronic bacterial prostatitis have no prior history of an acute prostatitis. Chills and fevers are unusual; dysuria, urgency, frequency and nocturia are common. There are no characteristic palpable prostatic findings in this disorder. Because adequate drug concentrations rarely are achieved in the prostatic secretions of these patients, the pathogen obtains sanctuary there; thus, the hallmark in diagnosis of chronic prostatitis is recurring urinary tract infections, always produced by the same pathogen. Infected prostatic calculi may or may not be associated with chronic bacterial prostatitis. Medical and manipulative management is the same as in acute bacterial prostatitis but the prognosis for complete "cure" is much poorer; surgical intervention is probably indicated for those with prostatic calculi.

Chronic non-bacterial prostatitis is more common than bacterial prostatitis; however, these patients rarely have histories of UTI and cultures fail to grow a pathogenic organism. Cells found in the prostatic secretions suggest an inflammatory component. Because the cause of non-bacterial prostatitis is "unknown," treatment is empirical, traditionally involving hot sitz baths and periodic prostatic massage. While these may prove helpful, the osteopathic approach adds manipulative treatment to correct any somatic dysfunction found in both the T12-L2 and S2-4 regions and to improve the function of the pelvic floor; the latter producing a physiologic "massage" of the prostate, occurring each time the patient takes a breath.

URETHRAL HYPERTONIA MAY LEAD TO OR BE CAUSED BY CHRONIC NONSPECIFIC PROSTATITIS (Adapted from Barbalias[34])

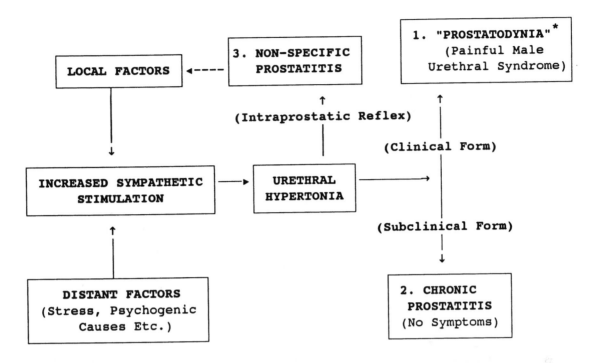

* Since prostatodynia literally means painful prostate, a better term to use might be "painful male urethral syndrome." In this syndrome, the increased urethral tone causes a painful urethra and not pain in the prostate (which in the over-whelming majority of these cases is nontender on palpation.)

Prostatodynia presents with variable pelvic pain, intermittent urgency, frequency, nocturia and dysuria as well as hesitancy and weakening of the urinary stream. Bacterial pathogens and inflammatory cells are not seen in the urine or prostatic expressate. Heightened sympathetic tone[34] and pelvic diaphragm tension[35] are reported to play a role in this symptom profile. The sympathetic dyssynergia causes spasm during voiding and seems to play a particularly significant role in patients with certain types of neurogenic obstruction.[36]

Recommended treatment would address the pelvic floor[37] and sympathetic mechanisms[38] involved as well as any postural, psychic, emotional or cultural stressors[39] which aggravate these mechanisms.

URETEROLITHIASIS (CALCULI):

Approximately 1/1000 adults annually will acutely suffer through the passage of at least one calculus through the ureter, bladder, and urethra. While many calculi are "silent", they typically produce excruciating pain in the thoracolumbar region radiating into common pain patterns in the back, lower abdomen, flank, and/or thigh.

Back pain or renal colic may occur with calculi in the calyces, renal pelvis, or upper ureter; while stones in the bladder may cause suprapubic pain.

Nausea, vomiting, abdominal distension, or the development of ileus are secondary gastrointestinal symptoms which may complicate or mask the correct diagnosis. Fever, chills, urinary frequency and hematuria are common signs and symptoms. Occasionally the ipsilateral kidney will reflexly and transiently become nonfunctional.

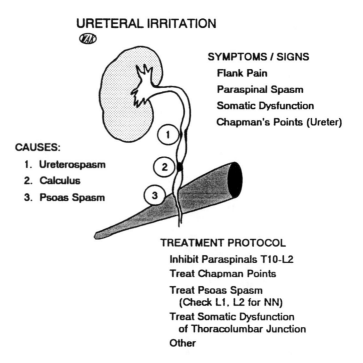

URETERAL IRRITATION

SYMPTOMS / SIGNS
Flank Pain
Paraspinal Spasm
Somatic Dysfunction
Chapman's Points (Ureter)

CAUSES:
1. Ureterospasm
2. Calculus
3. Psoas Spasm

TREATMENT PROTOCOL
Inhibit Paraspinals T10-L2
Treat Chapman Points
Treat Psoas Spasm
   (Check L1, L2 for NN)
Treat Somatic Dysfunction
   of Thoracolumbar Junction
Other

In cases with unilateral ureteral stones, the ipsilateral kidney becomes hypersensitive to emotional stress. Patients with unilateral renal disease demonstrate ipsilateral diminished renal blood flow and reduced GFR for 30-50 minutes.[40]

Predictable and predictive palpatory findings can be noted as the stone passes through the GU system. Because the pain is made worse and the passage of a calculus is slowed by ureterospasm, treatment considerations should include reduction of hypersympathicotonia through the use of thoracolumbar paraspinal inhibition and/or gentle rib raising techniques.

In the choice of pain medication, morphine should be avoided since this narcotic is more likely than demerol to produce an increase in smooth muscle spasm. Demerol does not cause significant ureteral smooth muscle contraction and is therefore a better pharmacologic choice for analgesia in this situation. The patient may appreciate paraspinal inhibition manipulation at the spinal level of reflex spasm until the demerol injection takes effect.

In cases of excruciating pain, most other OMT would be delayed until at least partial pain management has been achieved. When less pain is being experienced, the patient may benefit from counterstrain treatment of palpable anterior myofascial tender points including commonly seen genitourinary Chapman's reflex points and Jones' iliopsoas points.[41] Physiologic ureteral peristalsis should be assisted in all patients by diagnosing and treating the sacroiliacs as indicated. Also, the importance of adequate lymphatic drainage as a "safety valve" preventing complications and tissue damage has already been pointed out in the section on pathophysiology.

If the stone cannot be successfully passed, sonic disruption, cystoscopic basket extraction, or surgical removal may be necessary to reestablish normal function and prevent renal damage.

It is important to try to determine the pathogenesis of the stone so that proper prophylaxis can be planned to prevent recurrence. Fluids, dietary counselling, and modification of urinary pH along with a manipulative program designed to maintain or augment homeostatic GU mechanisms, can then be intelligently prescribed.

DYSMENORRHEA:

Primary dysmenorrhea should be differentiated from the many causes of secondary dysmenorrhea. The etiology of primary dysmenorrhea is unknown, but it occurs only with ovulatory cycles. This complaint of painful menstruation is quite common among young women. Both primary and secondary dysmenorrhea are aggravated by stress. An autonomic postural role has been implicated and the incidence of dysmenorrhea in college women is significantly greater in those with increased lumbar curvatures than in control populations.[42] An acutely anteverted cervix, in which the fundus is tipped anteriorly relative to the uterus, is one structural factor which is occasionally associated with dysmenorrhea. The cramp-like pain of dysmenorrhea is usually located in the lower abdomen but may include the back and thighs.

Treatment of any associated myofascial trigger points in the lower rectus abdominus will reduce symptoms of dysmenorrhea.[43] Dysmenorrhea may be associated with urinary frequency, pelvic soreness, abdominal distension, nausea, diarrhea, headache, depression, or irritability. Again, stress aggravates both primary and secondary dysmenorrhea as well as segmental facilitation and myofascial trigger points.

"Dysmenorrhea is one of the disorders in which osteopathic manipulative treatment (see chart on page 141) offers a great potential benefit."[44] The symptoms of primary dysmenorrhea are felt to arise from an imbalance in both the sympathetic and the parasympathetic systems as well as from somatic dysfunction causing a significant amount of venous and lymphatic congestion. Treatment to normalize both the sympathetics arising from T12-L2 (controlling uterine contraction and vasoconstriction) and the parasympathetics arising from S2-4 (controlling uterine inhibition and vasodilation) is a major goal; yet, this does not necessarily mean inhibiting one system and stimulating the other. Techniques to increase venous and lymphatic drainage of the pelvic organs often provides significant relief and is the other major goal of treatment.

One very effective manipulative technique used in accomplishing the goals outlined above involves a firm, continuous pressure over the sacral base with the patient in the prone position. This technique has an effect on the parasympathetics but is even more effective in fluid mobilization. The technique takes the sacral base anteriorly or into the "extension phase" of the craniosacral mechanism and is therefore equivalent to performing a CV4 cranial technique which is primarily used to help relieve tissue congestion in the body. Another technique that is effective in the acute phase is accomplished by gently rocking the prone patient's sacrum with its natural rhythm of 10-14 times a minute. This is postulated to improve the patient's parasympathetic outflow to the involved organs. Aspirin or NSAIDs may also be beneficial because they antagonize the spasmogenic action of prostaglandins and provide mild analgesia.

The monthly appearance of some cases of dysmenorrhea would benefit from monthly OMT to reduce the severity of symptoms. This is particularly true when they significantly impact the patient's abilities to participate in work, school, or home activities-of-daily-living. Functional dysmenorrhea may respond to an osteopathic manipulative approach which treats the functional cause. Osteopathic diagnosis and manipulative treatment may be clinically successful in relieving dysmenorrhea, particularly in the following situations:

o .. Using OMT and progressive heel lift treatment for correction of a short leg syndrome having a thoracolumbar cross-over and sacroiliac strain.
o .. Manipulation of craniosacral somatic dysfunction in a patient whose history reveals that the dysmenorrhea began after starting orthodontic treatment.
o .. Manipulation to remove a sacral shear in a teenage patient who reports that the dysmenorrhea began after a "pratfall". (Questioning the patient about specific activities such as roller skating, ice skating, and gymnastics can be very helpful in triggering the memory of significant trauma of this sort.)

The knee-chest position is used as an "exercise" which is frequently helpful in patients with dysmenorrhea. Requiring only 5-10 minutes to perform, this procedure is not a muscle strengthening exercise, but rather a body position to encourage optimal venous and lymphatic drainage from the pelvis and permit the uterus to lift out of the pelvis.

A PLAN FOR OSTEOPATHIC MANIPULATION OF A PATIENT WITH DYSMENORRHEA

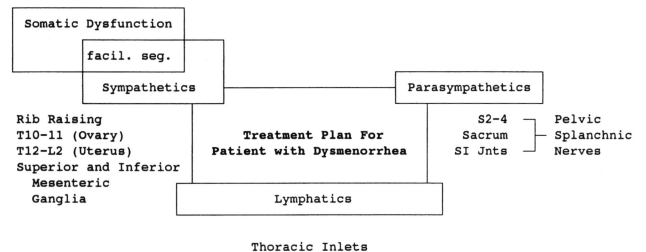

SYMPATHETIC (PATHO)PHYSIOLOGY (T10-11) and (T12-L2)

↑ Tone:

    1. ↑ Vasoconstriction → Poor Nutrition and O_2 Exchange
    2. ↑ Uterine Contractions
    3. ↓ Threshold for Pain (from uterine body)

LYMPHATIC (PATHO)PHYSIOLOGY

Impaired Lymphatic Flow:

    1. ↓ Lymph Flow
    2. ↑ Tissue Congestion → Bloating and Discomfort

PARASYMPATHETIC (PATHO)PHYSIOLOGY (S2,3,4)

↑ Tone:

    1. ↑ Relaxation of Uterine Muscle
    2. ↑ Vasodilation
    3. ↓ Threshold for Pain (from the cervix)

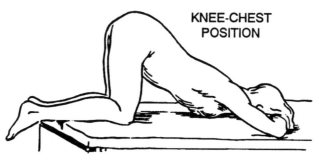

KNEE-CHEST
POSITION

Dorland WA, _The American Illustrated Medical Dictionary_,
Twenty-second edition, WB Saunders, 1951

With the patient resting her head and neck and chest down on her arms and with
her pelvis raised to a position just above her knees (the knee-chest position), the
abdominal contents will move with the pull of gravity out of the pelvis and
allow decongestion of the uterus. The patient may need to open the labia
momentarily to permit air into the vagina before the uterus moves. The patient
should do this exercise before retiring at night to obtain a maximal decongestive
effect.

SEXUAL DYSFUNCTION:

Proper sexual functioning involves a complex interaction of somatic,
parasympathetic, and sympathetic reflexes and the body unit tenet of the
osteopathic profession incorporating mental, emotional, and spiritual factors
which must be considered in this bodily function. Physiologic mechanisms
approximately parallel one another in men and women. Sexual dysfunction can
easily occur with imbalance in the autonomic nervous system, with negative
cortical influence, as well as with damage to neural, vascular or hormonal
mechanisms. OMT has been postulated to play a significant role in correcting
functional components of sexual dysfunction in several states including the
following:

o .. **ERECTILE DYSFUNCTION (IMPOTENCE):** At least half of the adult
   male population has experienced the inability to complete sexual
   intercourse in 25% or more of opportunities because of erectile
   dysfunction. Psychic factors are usually the cause; however, other
   functional disorders may play a significant role in this problem.
   Erection is dependent upon somatic input through the pudendal nerve
   (S2-4) and parasympathetic reflexes (S2-4) and therefore manipulative
   treatment to remove any sacroiliac somatic dysfunction may be helpful
   when organic reasons have been ruled out.

In the female, the physiologic equivalent would be dysfunction of arousal and lubrication. These conditions may also play a role in development of frigidity and/or dyspareunia.

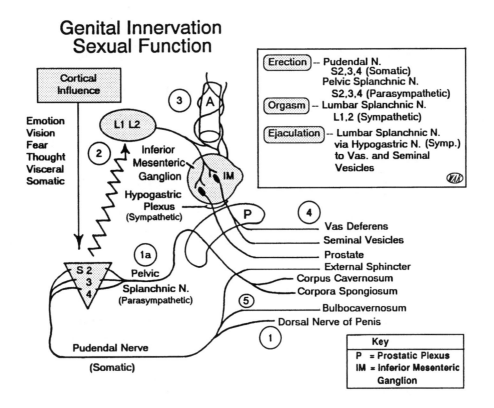

Genital Innervation
Sexual Function

Erection -- Pudendal N.
S2,3,4 (Somatic)
Pelvic Splanchnic N.
S2,3,4 (Parasympathetic)
Orgasm -- Lumbar Splanchnic N.
L1,2 (Sympathetic)
Ejaculation -- Lumbar Splanchnic N.
via Hypogastric N. (Symp.)
to Vas. and Seminal
Vesicles

Cortical Influence

Emotion
Vision
Fear
Thought
Visceral
Somatic

L1 L2

Inferior Mesenteric Ganglion

Hypogastric Plexus (Sympathetic)

Pelvic Splanchnic N. (Parasympathetic)

Pudendal Nerve

(Somatic)

Vas Deferens
Seminal Vesicles
Prostate
External Sphincter
Corpus Cavernosum
Corpora Spongiosum
Bulbocavernosum
Dorsal Nerve of Penis

Key	
P	= Prostatic Plexus
IM	= Inferior Mesenteric Ganglion

o .. **PREMATURE EJACULATION:** Ejaculation is primarily a sympathetically-mediated event activated through L1-2 and aided by somatic influence from S2-4. Osteopathic manipulation to somatic dysfunctions in the L1-2 area of the spine and efforts to reduce visceral afferent information to L1-2 (i.e. treatment for left colon or pelvic disorders) may help a patient who is having this type of ejaculation dysfunction. OMT to these areas reduces facilitation to the L1-2 sympathetic centers in the spinal cord. Educating the patient to interrupt sensory input from the penis and/or L1-2 dermatomes prior to orgasm and ejaculation is also helpful.

o .. **DYSPAREUNIA:** This condition may arise from spasm of the vagina, inadequate lubrication, pelvic floor spasm, or lesions and abnormalities of the female genital tract. The success of osteopathic treatment in patients with this problem is related to the correction of somatic dysfunction which affects the attachments of the pelvic diaphragm and normalize parasympathetic reflex activity permitting formation of adequate vaginal lubrication. In the atrophic vagina, estrogen creams may be helpful.

o .. **INFERTILITY:** Approximately 10% of married couples in the United States have infertility. Because fertility requires function and coordination of the physiologic mechanisms of two individuals, there is a great potential for a dysfunctional cause of infertility. Female structural tubal disorders are only accountable for 30% of the cases. Male gonadal deficiency accounts for 40%, female hormonal deficiency 20%, and "hostile" cervical environment 10%.

Because of cost, mental duress, and time involved in the investigation of infertility, the osteopathic general practice approach incorporates a therapeutic trial of OMT, education, reassurance and correction of any structural, infectious, or emotional stresses which might interfere with correct functioning. Structurally, emphasis is placed on normalizing thoracolumbar and pelvic somatic dysfunction and reducing postural disorders which might be involved in perpetuating segmental facilitation. Craniosacral evaluation and treatment to assure that there is no functional pituitary-ovarian axis problem are also considered beneficial.

Couples in which irregular menstrual cycles were a complicating factor often report they had increased opportunity for better and less stressful timing of the critical period of ovulation and conception after OMT promoted regularized periods. Preliminary studies have suggested an elevation in previously low spermatic counts following systemic OMT.[45] Certainly there is a general reduction in stress which, when coupled with the removal of somatic and visceral components of "the neurologic lens" (segmental facilitation), offers improved physiologic function. This approach has often rewarded the couple with clinical success, a long-awaited pregnancy.[46]

An infertility workup becomes necessary only when there is failure of a clinical therapeutic trial of osteopathic management over a reasonable length of time. This program must be individually designed to treat infections and rule out other organic disease, maximize the patients' own reproductive function and create a favorable environment for implantation and fetal growth.

ADDITIONAL GENITOURINARY BIBLIOGRAPHY:

Goldthwait, Brown, Swain, Kulans Essentials of Body Mechanics in Health and Disease. 5th ed, 1952.

Winter CC Practical Urology. Mosby Co, 1969.

Pottenger FM Symptoms of Visceral Disease. St Louis, CV Mosby Co, 7th ed, 1953.

Szwed JJ et al: The effect of IV mannitol on renal hemodynamics and renal lymph recovery during acute ureteral obstruction , in Foldi (ed) Progress in Lymphology. 1967, pp 123-26.

REFERENCE:

1. Sterrett HW, Jr: Disorders of the urinary system, in Hoag JM (ed) Osteopathic Medicine. New York, McGraw-Hill, 1969, ch 40, p 657.
2. Goldthwait, Brown, Swain, Kuhns Essentials of Body Mechanics in Health and Disease. 5th ed, 1952.
3. Ibid
4. Hix EL: Viscerovisceral and somatovisceral reflex communications, in Korr IM (ed), The Physiological Basis of Osteopathic Medicine, New York, Insight Publ Company Inc, 1975, pp 87-8.
5. Ibid
6. Op cit p 89.
7. Daiber WF: Disorders of the kidneys, in Hoag JM (ed) Osteopathic Medicine. New York, McGraw-Hill, 1969, ch 39, p 640.
8. Awad SA, Downie JW: Sympathetic dyssynergia in the region of the external sphincter: A possible source of lower urinary tract obstruction. Journal of Urology 1977; 118:636-640.
9. Barbalias GA, Meares EM, Sant GR: Prostatodynia: Clinical and urodynamic characteristics. Journal of Urology 1983; 130:514-517.
10. Guyton Textbook of Physiology.
11. Owens C An Endocrine Interpretation of Chapman's Reflexes. Carmel CA, 1963.
12. Awad SA, Downie JW: Sympathetic dyssynergia in the region of the external sphincter: A possible source of lower urinary tract obstruction. Journal of Urology 1977; 118:636-640.
13. Saunders JB: The major determinants in normal and pathological gait. Journal of Bone and Joint Surgery Jul 1953; 35-A(3): 543-558.
14. Segura JW, Opitz JL, and Greene LF: Prostatosis, prostatitis or pelvic floor tension myalgia? Journal of Urology 1979: 122:168-169.
15. Sterrett HW, Jr: Disorders of the urinary system, in Hoag JM (ed) Osteopathic Medicine. New York, McGraw-Hill, 1969, ch 40, p 664.
16. Sinaki M, Merritt JL, Sillwell GK: Tension myalgia of the pelvic floor. Mayo Clin Proc 1977; 52:717-722.
17. Travell JG, Simons DG Myofascial Pain and Dysfunction: A Trigger Point Manual, Baltimore, Williams & Wilkins, 1983, p 671.
18. Ibid
19. Burrows EA: Disorders of the female reproductive system, in Hoag JM Osteopathic Medicine. New York, McGraw-Hill, 1969, ch 42, p 681.
20. Op cit p 677.

21. Pottenger FM <u>Symptoms of Visceral Disease</u>. St Louis, CV Mosby Co, 1953, 7th ed, p 401.
22. Dobrik I: Disorders of the iliopsoas muscle and its role in gynecologic diseases. <u>J Manual Med</u> 1989; 4(4): 130-133.
23. Ibid
24. Ibid
25. Travell JG, Simons DG <u>Myofascial Pain and Dysfunction: A Trigger Point Manual</u>. Baltimore, Williams & Wilkins, 1983, p 665.
26. Burrows EA: Disorders of the female reproductive system, in Hoag JM <u>Osteopathic Medicine</u>. New York, McGraw-Hill, 1969, ch 42, p 678.
27. Daiber WF: Disorders of the kidneys, in Hoag JM (ed) <u>Osteopathic Medicine</u>. New York, McGraw-Hill, 1969, ch 39, p 634.
28. Op cit p 639.
29. Ibid
30. Sterrett HW, Jr: Disorders of the urinary system, in Hoag JM (ed) <u>Osteopathic Medicine</u>. New York, McGraw-Hill, 1969, ch 40, p 663.
31. Op cit p 661.
32. Op cit pp 663-664.
33. Drach GW, Fair WR, Meares EM and Stamey TA: Classification of benign diseases associated with prostatic pain: Prostatitis or prostatodynia? <u>Journal of Urology</u> 1978; 120:266.
34. Barbalias GA, Meares EM, and Sant GR: Prostatodynia: Clinical and urodynamic characteristics. <u>Journal of Urology</u> 1983; 130:514-517.
35. Sinaki M, Merritt JL, Sillwell GK: Tension myalgia of the pelvic floor. <u>Mayo Clin Proc</u> 1977; 52:717-722.
36. Awad SA, Downie JW: Sympathetic dyssynergia in the region of the external sphincter: A possible source of lower urinary tract obstruction. <u>Journal of Urology</u>, 1977; 118:636-640.
37. Segura JW, Opitz JL, Greene LF: Prostatosis, prostatitis of pelvic floor tension myalgia? <u>Journal of Urology</u> 1979; 122: 168-169.
38. Awad SA, Downie JW: Sympathetic dyssenergia in the region of the external sphincter: A possible source of lower urinary tract obstruction. <u>Journal of Urology</u> 1977; 118: 636-640.
39. Nilsson IK, Colleen S, Mardh PA: Relationship between psychological and laboratory findings in patients with symptoms of non-acute prostatitis, in Danielsson D, Juhlin L, and Mardh PA (eds) <u>Genital Infections and Their Complications</u>. Stockholm, Almquist and Wiksell Intl, 1975, pp 133-144.
40. Hix EL: Viscerovisceral and somatovisceral reflex communication, in Korr IM (ed), <u>The Physiologic Basis of Osteopathic Manipulation</u>. New York, Insight Publishing Co, Inc, 1975, p. 91.
41. Jones L <u>Strain and Counterstrain</u>. AAO, Colorado Springs, 1981.
42. Jenness M: The role of thermography and postural measurement in structural diagnosis, in Goldstein M, <u>The Research Status of Spinal Manipulative Therapy</u>. Bethesda MD, US Department of Health Education and Welfare (NINCDS Monograph #15) 1975, p 258.
43. Travell JG, Simons DG <u>Myofascial Pain and Dysfunction: A Trigger Point Manual</u>. Baltimore, Williams & Wilkins, 1983, p 665.

44. Burrows EA: Disorders of the female reproductive system, in Hoag JM (ed) <u>Osteopathic Medicine</u>. New York, McGraw-Hill, 1969, ch 42, p 682.

45. Sterrett HW, Jr: Disorders of the male genitourinary system, in Hoag JM (ed) <u>Osteopathic Medicine</u>. New York, McGraw-Hill, 1969, ch 41, p 673.
   and G Slattery, DO, PhD -- unpublished case history, KCOM.

46. Ibid (Sterrett)
   and Burrows EA: Disorders of the female reproductive system, in Hoag JM (ed) <u>Osteopathic Medicine</u>. New York, McGraw-Hill, 1969, ch 42, p 678.

NOTES:

OSTEOPATHIC CONSIDERATIONS IN THE OBSTETRICAL PATIENT

"It is physiologically imperative that we provide for optimal growth and development of the fetus while preserving the maternal homeostasis." Although expressed by Dr. Roy Pitkin, an obstetrician from The Iowa University School of Medicine who is noted for his knowledge of nutrition in the OB patient, this also sums up the osteopathic perspective applied in obstetrics. Total care for the obstetrical patient is a physician's desire regardless of his medical degree; however, a physician's ability to provide total care to the patient is, in fact, a variable.

I. EXISTING STRESSES AGGRAVATED BY PREGNANCY

GRAVITY:

o .. Gravity mainly affects the A-P postural curves aggravating lumbar and cervical lordoses and thoracic kyphosis..

o .. Gravity, activity, habits and stresses of motion produce fascial torsions.

o .. The normal aging process amplifies the effects of gravity and/or fascial torsions.

A BASIC PHYSIOLOGICAL RELATIONSHIP: More blood gets to the tissues than can be returned by the venous system.

Blood gets to the cells via the arteries and into the interstitial spaces through the capillaries. The interstitial tissue fluids get back to the heart via the venous system with necessary and vital assistance from the lymphatic system (which has no intrinsic pump).

o .. More blood gets to the tissues than can be removed by the venous system; therefore the lymphatic system is essential if tissue congestion is to be prevented--in fact, it is essential for life itself.

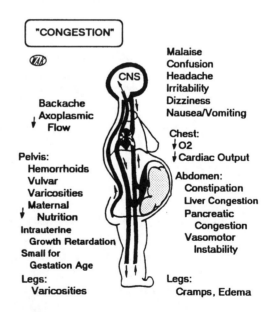

"CONGESTION"

CNS

Malaise
Confusion
Headache
Irritability
Dizziness
Nausea/Vomiting

Backache
↓ Axoplasmic
Flow

Chest:
↓ O2
↓ Cardiac Output

Pelvis:
Hemorrhoids
Vulvar
Varicosities
↓ Maternal
Nutrition
Intrauterine
Growth Retardation
Small for
Gestation Age

Abdomen:
Constipation
Liver Congestion
Pancreatic
Congestion
Vasomotor
Instability

Legs:
Varicosities

Legs:
Cramps, Edema

Anything which increases circulation to the cells will result in increased interstitial tissue fluids and result in increased demands upon the

lymphatic system to move these fluids in order to prevent tissue
congestion or edema.

o .. The abdominal diaphragm functions as an "extrinsic" pump for the
lymphatic system. When working well, it produces effective pressure
gradients between the chest and the abdominal cavities. The pressure
gradients, along with the valves in the larger lymphatic vessels, produce
a most effective force for the one-way flow of lymph back to the venous
system and the heart. Sympathetic impulses are capable of constricting
larger lymphatic vessels; therefore, hypersympathetic tone is a factor
which decreases lymph flow and promotes tissue congestion.

**THE UNIQUE VALVELESS VENOUS SYSTEM: The CNS, spinal cord
and the bony vertebral column contain a "valveless venous system."**

Physiological factors working upon the valveless venous system of the spine
have the ability to produce patterns of flow which result in venous congestion in
the tissues they are supposed to drain, decrease organ function and generally
increase a person's level of stress.

o .. Because there are no valves in these venous plexuses, blood is free to move
in either direction depending upon the path of least resistance.

o .. About 80% of the blood from the brain and its meninges exits the jugular
foramina of the skull by way of the jugular veins. Blood from the spinal
cord, its membranes, and the bony vertebral column (the spine) usually
passes through communicating veins, to enter the veins of the azygos and
hemiazygos system. The communicating veins are also valveless and not
consistently present at each lumbar and thoracic level. The venous blood
from these areas usually drains into the heart via the superior vena cava.

A secondary pathway for drainage of the profuse venous plexuses of the
spinal cord and vertebral system is provided through anastomoses of
these plexuses with the vertebral and the internal jugular veins at the
base of the skull.

o .. Venous blood in this closed system is "pushed" by the arterial blood volume
propelled by the contractions of the heart and pulled by pressure
gradients largely arising from respiratory efforts. The amount and
proportion of venous blood which travels through the valveless
communicating veins or through the anastomoses with the vertebral and
internal jugular veins is affected by any change in the resting pressure in
the thorax or abdomen; flow through this secondary route is also
increased by any decrease in the gradient of pressure between the
abdominal and thoracic cavities. These physical factors can produce

150

flow dynamics which lead to relative congestion in the CNS, the spinal membranes and/or the bony vertebral spine.

II. STRESSES ADDED SPECIFICALLY BY PREGNANCY

Stresses of a normal pregnancy produce a relatively rapid aging process which is usually reversible. These stresses are produced through mechanical, physiological, venous/lymphatic and hormonal changes.

MECHANICAL: The musculoskeletal system and the body's center of gravity is changed.

Organ hypertrophy and mechanical stress produce structural change and a shift in the body's center of gravity. The changes brought about by mechanical stress are accelerated by the effect of circulating hormones of pregnancy which tend to weaken muscle and supporting ligaments.

It has been shown that dysfunction in the musculoskeletal system can increase the energy requirements of an individual up to 300%.

PHYSIOLOGICAL: Interstitial fluids are increased.

Additional production of interstitial fluids is brought about by the increased circulation necessary to meet the additional metabolic demands of the growing fetus and placenta and to support the hypertrophy of the uterus and other organs. Increased levels of estrogen and adrenal hormones also promote fluid retention in the body's tissues.

LYMPHATIC: There is decreased efficiency in the removal of excessive interstitial fluids.

Fascial torsions hinder the flow of lymph through lymphatic vessels travelling through the connective tissues; organ hypertrophy and downward drag of the abdominal wall produce volume changes in the abdomen and thorax; structural stresses (increased lumbar lordotic curves, thoracic kyphotic curves, tension on the diaphragm, and anterior sacral base) and the downward drag of the abdominal and thoracic wall may act singly or in concert to promote poor diaphragmatic excursion. All of these factors decrease the diaphragm's ability to produce the most effective pressure gradients necessary to promote good lymphatic flow and to reduce tissue congestion. It is clinically observed that generalized symptoms of lymphatic and venous congestion present as clinical problems, especially in the last trimester of a patient's prenatal care.

VENOUS: There is a tendency for venous congestion of the central nervous system (CNS).

There is a drastic change in the volume of organs which occupy the abdomen as well as changes in the relative volume and pressure gradients between the abdominal and thoracic cavities. These changes tend to increase the cavity pressures and encourage a relative reversal of venous blood flow in the valveless communicating, vertebral and spinal membrane vessels and lead to relative congestion of the central nervous system (CNS). Symptoms of venous congestion are more evident in the early part of the first trimester, the last trimester, and in the postpartum period.

HORMONAL: Increases in hormone production encourage tissue congestion.

Increased levels of certain hormones during pregnancy promote biological weakening of muscles and ligaments and encourage fluid retention. These changes then permit a focusing of mechanical stress onto certain biomechanically sensitive areas of the body, reducing effectiveness of the diaphragm's lymphatic pump action, and directly increasing interstitial fluids while at the same time promoting changes which result in obstruction of lymphatic pathways back to the heart.

RELATIVE CONTRAINDICATIONS TO OMT:

While OMT can be helpful in pre-eclampsia, the seizure threshold is low in toxemia of pregnancy and OMT is seldom a part of a treatment protocol. OMT is also usually avoided during premature rupture of membranes, premature labor, abruptio placentae, and ectopic pregnancies.

III. DISTINCTIVE OSTEOPATHIC THINKING:

Distinctive osteopathic thinking to improve the compensation and comfort of the OB patient is based upon three premises:

o .. There are mechanical, physiological and biological stresses inherent even in the patient who is destined to have a normal pregnancy.
o .. The body has self-regulatory mechanisms which will provide optimal compensation for the stresses of pregnancy if they are free to work efficiently.
o .. Distinctive osteopathic care is based upon the belief and the clinical observations that within the body unit, structure and function are reciprocally interrelated and interwoven with optimum homeostasis.

AN AID IN PREVENTIVE CARE: Postural analysis and palpatory examination early in pregnancy can identify areas of somatic dysfunction which, if uncorrected, act to focus the stresses of pregnancy on vulnerable sites within the body unit.

A DIAGNOSTIC AID: Both visceral and structural dysfunction are indicated by palpable changes in the somatic structures.

A TREATMENT ADVANTAGE: Proper osteopathic manipulative treatment to the areas of structural dysfunction is associated with improvement of visceral and somatic function.

IV. DISTINCTIVE OSTEOPATHIC TREATMENT:

Any licensed physician who accepts the care of obstetrical patients should have been trained to take care of her medical and delivery needs. In addition to this, an osteopathic physician is trained to appreciate and treat the musculoskeletal and physiological stresses which occur in pregnancy. Manipulative treatment normalizes somatic dysfunction which produces and/or focuses mechanical stress. It also improves the efficiency of mechanical and physiologic components of the patient's compensatory and homeostatic processes. The energy that is subsequently saved through improved body efficiency and removal of somatic dysfunction will be available for fetal growth and for the betterment of maternal physical and mental health.

"THE STRUCTURAL STAGE:" First visit to 28th week of gestation -- Monthly visits:

0-12 WEEKS:

The patient usually makes her first visit during the 9th-12th week of pregnancy and although she has experienced some of the early signs and symptoms of pregnancy, her structure is little affected at this stage. During these first three months, the patient normally gains about 2.5 to 4.5 pounds.

At the patient's first visit the physician obtains a complete history including the history of past pregnancies, deliveries, family history of significant diseases, and asks about habits--smoking, coffee, alcohol or the use of drugs. If drugs have been used it is important to know if the patient has stopped them--and if so, how long ago. The physician should find out about the patient's eating habits.

At the first visit the physician establishes rapport with the patient and the patient establishes a lasting impression of her physician. This is important, but is not unique to osteopathic care. The remainder of this chapter will try to highlight the osteopathic differences in management.

The osteopathic physician is very interested in any history of past accidents to the head or the rest of the musculoskeletal system. This includes car accidents, blows to the head, falls down the stairs, or falls on the buttocks. This may be just routine information in most medical histories but, to the osteopathic physician, a positive response to any of these questions must be investigated. These stresses may have resulted in persistent somatic dysfunction which could affect the patient's ability to effectively compensate for the stress of pregnancy.

The patient is asked if she has any present musculoskeletal complaints. During the routine physical, palpatory evidence of these and other somatic dysfunctions and structural abnormalities such as a short leg, a sacral shear, or scoliosis is sought.

o .. In the standing position quickly observe and record the levelness of the various regional horizontal planes--occipital, shoulder, iliac crests, PSIS, and trochanteric. The spine is observed and palpated for rotoscoliosis as the patient bends forward at the waist.

o .. In the sitting position the preference for fascial motion at the thoracic inlet can be quickly assessed to see whether it is symmetrical or whether it conforms (or not) to the common compensatory pattern as described by the late Dr. Gordon Zink. A problem with the fascial inlet patterns must be differentiated from the somewhat similar findings of an elevated 1st rib somatic dysfunction. The ribs and the thoracic and lumbar spine can also be evaluated for segmental somatic dysfunction in the sitting position.

At this time the physician may manipulate any somatic dysfunction that has been identified. (The sitting or standing pillow technique--utilizing a pillow to localize the thrust--is very helpful in treating the pregnant patient, even during the third trimester.

o .. With the patient in the supine position, the rest of the regional fascial patterning (OA, thoracolumbar and lumbosacral) can be evaluated and the pelvis can be palpated for somatic dysfunction (SD) of the innominates or pubic bones. The physician usually proceeds to treat the SD found in these areas, using any osteopathic manipulative technique tolerated by the patient. Most techniques which would be performed in a patient who is not pregnant can be used in the pregnant patient at this stage of her pregnancy.

o .. In the prone position (an easy position to assume during this early part of pregnancy) the sacrum can be evaluated and treated as indicated. A sacral shear (a non-physiological somatic dysfunction) must be removed or the patient will be assured of having backaches during pregnancy and manipulative treatments for other somatic dysfunction will not have a lasting effect.

o .. Finally, have the patient assume the supine position again and check the cervical spine and the craniosacral mechanism by palpation and motion testing. Any somatic dysfunction in these regions should be treated at this time.

From the history, physical examination, and her subjective and tissue response to treatment, the physician can determine the osteopathic manipulative care necessary, the probable dosage indicated, and what the manipulative treatments should be able to accomplish before delivery.

12-28 WEEKS:

During the second half of the structural stage, the physician still sees the patient at monthly intervals, although if indicated, more frequent appointments are provided. A little extra time now will save a lot of time and worry later on in the pregnancy. At each visit, part of the care is directed toward manipulation of SD (which may be a part of her complaints) and/or part toward manipulative support of body structures and processes which the osteopathic physician knows will be under stress. This treatment is easily carried out as the patient talks to the physician and the physician talks to her. "The time to talk to each other" is extremely important to the patient/doctor relationship and to mutual trust.

It is known that during the structural stage (the second trimester), there will be obvious changes in her body structure--increased fat storage, growth of the uterus, hypertrophy of the breast and other tissues, blood volume expansion, and a shift in the patient's center of gravity. The pelvis will rock forward, lumbar lordosis will increase, and a compensatory thoracic kyphosis will develop along with a cervical/suboccipital strain. Near the end of this first stage (second trimester), clinical evidence of tissue congestion may begin to appear.

Muscles and ligaments become more vulnerable to the mechanical stresses as biological effects of increased levels of hormones weaken their strength. These structural effects of stress are often subjective and are usually very obvious to the osteopathic physician.

"THE CONGESTIVE STAGE:" Visits Every 3 Weeks:

28-36TH WEEK:

This part of the pregnancy is called the "congestive phase." Congestion occurs when more fluid accumulates in the tissues than can be effectively removed by the venous and lymphatic systems. This congestion is partly mechanical, partly hormonal, and partly biological. Circulating hormones, in increased amounts, have the tendency to encourage the body to hold water in the tissues. The patient's symptoms vary depending upon which tissues become congested. Tissue congestion is also associated with decreased oxygenation and nutrition of the cells and is related to increased accumulation of metabolites in the soft tissues.

During this stage of pregnancy, the expanding uterus is well above the umbilicus and is pushing toward the xiphoid process. It causes a mechanical, "ball-valve," effect between the veins of the legs and their abdominal connection with the inferior vena cava, and is mechanically responsible for some of the leg edema of late pregnancy. It also makes it difficult for some women to lie supine without becoming hypotensive. The uterus also pushes up under the diaphragm and the lower ribs. This limits the chest volume that can be obtained during respiration and directly affects the thoracic:abdominal pressure gradients which can be obtained.

The diaphragm must also work harder against the increased mass of abdominal and pelvic contents and this results in its increased tone. The diaphragm at this stage of the pregnancy is unable to produce optimal volume displacements between the thorax and the abdomen during contraction and relaxation and is associated with inefficiency in pumping the lymph back to the heart. A greater volume displacement is achieved through correction of thoracoabdominal and pelvic floor dysfunction.

Although the physician must continue to be alert for mechanical decompensation and treat to maintain good structure during this second stage as indicated, it is most important to check the common compensatory pattern (CCP) in order to maintain freedom of the fascial pathways and thus improve lymphatic drainage. (See page 207) Osteopathic manipulative treatment is directed toward maintaining symmetry of the thoracic inlet, relaxing the thoracolumbar junction (attachment of the abdominal diaphragm), and keeping the diaphragm well domed. After OMT, the abdomen feels softer and more mobile and diaphragmatic excursion is fuller. This type of treatment improves the efficiency of the thoracoabdominal pump and therefore improves lymphatic flow. Lymphatic flow can be "encouraged" by the use of the pectoralis lift technique (see page 230). The usual manipulative "chest pumps" may be uncomfortable because of hypertrophy and increased sensitivity of the breasts.

"THE PREPARATORY STAGE:" 36 WEEKS TO DELIVERY -- Weekly visits:

This is the final stage of pre-delivery care. If the patient ever expresses a feeling of "really being pregnant," this is the time. During this third stage of prenatal care, it is necessary to continue to maintain good structural balance and to support lymphatic flow, but it is imparative to emphasize two additional areas of care for the obstetrical patient:

o .. Begin to build the psychological support that the patient will need for delivery. Emphasize the positive points in her prenatal experience and help her to plan for the delivery.
o .. Carefully check the craniosacral mechanism to be sure it has a normal configuration, rate, and amplitude so that it will aid normal hormonal and neural function during labor and delivery.

If the osteopathic physician has been able to accomplish the goals presented to this point, the labor and delivery will usually go smoothly. If complications should occur, the patient is in better condition to compensate and reach a new homeostatic level.

"LABOR AND DELIVERY:"

OMT is infrequently used during the delivery itself; however, sacral pressure is frequently comforting during labor and can be taught to the husband to be performed periodically or at his wife's request. The physician may elect to use CV4 technique in postdate gravida women to induce uterine contraction[1] or to overcome uterine inertia during labor.

"THE RECOVERY AND MAINTENANCE STAGE:" Delivery to 6 weeks postpartum -- 2 visits:

o .. On the second day postpartum, the patient should be taken to the treatment room where a screening structural examination and indicated manipulative treatment is performed. The physician can use soft tissue, muscle energy, indirect, Jones counterstrain, cranial methods and even thrust manipulation, as needed.

The effects of circulating maternal hormones are still evident in the articular and ligamentous structures making treatment methods easier. Successful manipulation places the joints in good functional position as the hormonal effect wears off and the ligaments begin to return to their normal tension and strength.

During this stage of treatment the physician is still interested in treating the patient to improve lymphatic flow. Breast engorgement which occurs on the second day in the multipara and on the third day in the primipara is probably hormonal in etiology, but clinical experience indicates that patients with good lymphatic flow tend to have decreased complaints of breast congestion and a reduced incidence of the "postpartum blues."

Careful check of the sacrum during this early postpartum treatment session is essential. The mechanical progression of the infant through the birth canal and the lithotomy position of the patient during delivery encourages anterior sacral base somatic dysfunction and the extension phase of the craniosacral mechanism. It has been observed that significant anterior sacral base somatic dysfunction is associated with patient complaints of fatigue, depression, and low energy. The mechanical etiology of these symptoms can be avoided if the physician finds and treats this somatic dysfunction early and effectively.

o .. The usual final "OB" visit is at 6 weeks postpartum. The patient's progress up to this point is evaluated and a gyn/pap smear is repeated. If the obstetrical patient is treated as outlined, it is not common to find any specific somatic dysfunction to treat and the patient presents herself as being well and happy. This is the time to make sure she has a contraceptive program if desired, realizes the importance of self-breast exam and yearly gyn/pap smears, understands the importance of (and has an appointment for) a follow-up visit regarding any chronic problems that require further care. Osteopathic manipulative care is a part of the total care of the obstetrical patient. Its inclusion makes the prenatal time and delivery more comfortable for the patient, enforces a quicker and more complete recovery from delivery, and enhances this wonderful miraculous event of life.

REFERENCES:

1. Gitlin RS, Wolf DL: Uterine contractions following osteopathic cranial manipulation -- A pilot study. JAOA 92(9):1183, Sept 1992.

2. Zink JG, Lawson WG: Pressure gradients in the osteopathic manipulative management of the obstetrical patient. Osteopathic Annals May 1979; 7(5): 208-214.

3. Zink JG, Lawson WG: An osteopathic structural examination and functional interpretation of the soma. Osteopathic Annals Dec 1979; 7(12): 433-440.

4. Kuchera WA: Osteopathic considerations in the obstetrical patient. FAAO Thesis 1989.

5. Saunders JB et al: The major determinants in normal and pathological gait. Journal of Bone and Joint Surgery Jul 1953; 35-A(3): 543-558.

6. Pitkin RM: Assessment of nutritional status of mother, fetus, and newborn. The American Journal of Clinical Nutrition Apr 1981; 34: 658-668.

7. Heckman JD: Managing musculoskeletal problems in pregnant patients, part I. The Journal Of Musculoskeletal Medicine June 1984: 14-24.

8. Dilts PV, Jr, Gerbie, Sciarra: Exercise and physical activity during pregnancy, in Shrock P (ed) Gynecology And Obstetrics. Philadelphia, Harper And Row, vol 2, rev ed, 1985, ch 8.

OSTEOPATHIC CONSIDERATIONS
IN RHEUMATOLOGIC DISORDERS

I. INTRODUCTION

Osteopathic manipulative treatment (OMT) is an extremely valuable component in the care of a patient with a rheumatologic condition. While the adjective, "rheumatologic", denotes a joint musculoskeletal disorder, many rheumatologic disorders such as rheumatoid arthritis (RA) are chronic systemic diseases. By indirectly reducing the side effects of medications, directly enhancing homeostatic mechanisms, and maximizing function within the patient's existing structure, osteopathic palpatory diagnosis and manipulative treatment play special roles in the management of chronic illnesses. This section will focus primarily on the rationale for OMT in a patient with rheumatoid arthritis, but the rationale can be extended to other rheumatologic conditions.

II. PATHOPHYSIOLOGY

Articular cartilage is avascular, therefore its nutrition needs to be considered in any discussion of the pathogenesis of rheumatologic disease. Synovial fluid provides the joint access to nutrients as well as serving as a site for the disposal of metabolic wastes and immune complexes. In addition, the efficacy of any prescribed anti-inflammatory medications is dependent on their concentration in the synovial fluids. The transference of nutrients and medications into the synovial fluid and of immune complexes and other wastes out is dependent on diffusion. For this reason, factors affecting diffusion such as blood flow, concentration of nutrients and waste products in the region, and synovial membrane permeability are extremely relevant.

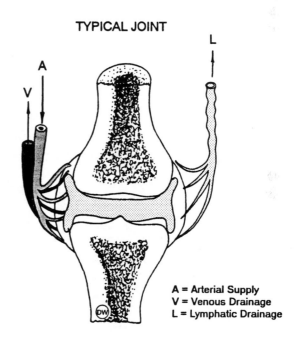

TYPICAL JOINT

A = Arterial Supply
V = Venous Drainage
L = Lymphatic Drainage

On the basis of histologic studies, cartilage is best preserved in those parts of the joint where the articular surface is subjected to intermittent compressive contact. This type of contact improves local nutrition of the cartilage and mobilizes immune complexes from the area. Accumulation of immune complexes is associated with increased joint destruction.

SYMPATHETICS:

In joints with rheumatoid arthritis, oxygen consumption is increased up to twenty times the amount used by a normal synovial membrane. Increased sympathetic activity further compromises blood flow to the involved joint(s) and reduces the delivery of nutrients (including oxygen) and medication to the area where it is needed the most. Tissue hypoxia may result in the release of polymorphonuclear leukocytes which promote multilamination of the basement membrane. This thickening further diminishes diffusion into and out of the synovial fluid of the joint.

AUTONOMIC NERVOUS SYSTEM: ROLE IN RHEUMATOLOGY

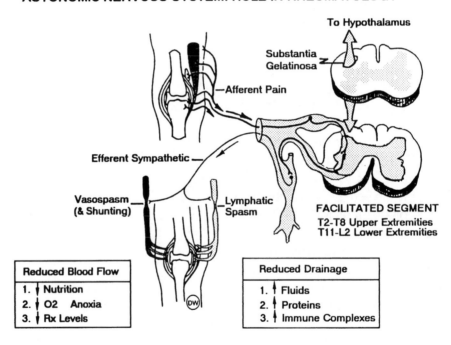

Because structure and function are interrelated and because rheumatoid arthritis alters joint structure, it should not be surprising that arthritis leads to the development of somatic dysfunction. Continuous afferent input to the cord from a dysfunctional joint incites facilitation in those cord segments. The flare-up of a patient's arthritic joint with resultant segmental spinal cord facilitation is

160

often accompanied by dysfunction of the viscera that share sympathetic innervation from those cord segments. This relationship can also be reversed, i.e. certain visceral diseases are associated with arthritic complications. The relationship of arthritis in the spine and lower extremity in patients with colitis is a common example of this relationship. The somatic innervation and somatic afferent referral to the spinal cord from the lower extremities are located from T11-L2 while the sympathetic innervation to the colon is also found from T10-L2. Likewise, increased afferent input from upper extremity joints to the T2-T8 sections of the spinal cord may reflexly increase the sympathetic activity to the upper gastrointestinal tract (T5-9) leading to reduced tolerance of the non-steroidal anti-inflammatory drugs (NSAIDs) used in the treatment of arthritis.

The sympathetic nervous system is capable of augmenting the symptomatology and pathogenesis of rheumatoid arthritis. Increased sympathetic activity sensitizes the patient's perception of pain both peripherally and centrally and plays a role in the muscle spasm and contracture that limits range of motion and intensifies deformity. Noxious somatic input reflexly sets up pathophysiologic change which bring about symptoms and signs which, carried to extreme, may result in a diagnosis of reflex sympathetic dystrophy (RSD). The sympathetic hyperactivity in this condition is also involved in initiating the bony erosion seen in joints of patients with rheumatoid arthritis. It has been reported that there is hypersympathetic activity in patients with RA, RSD and osteoporosis and that bilateral sympathectomy often helps limit bony erosion significantly in these patients.

Kelley's Textbook of Rheumatology states that even in the most aggressive cases of RA, only minimal reversible change occurs until after the lesion becomes chronic. "Chronicity" seems to take eight or more weeks. This information suggests a timeframe during which treatment directed toward the sympathetic nervous system may result in prevention by addressing reversible functional changes before they become structural.

SOMATIC SYSTEM:

Somatic dysfunction plays a role in the pathogenesis of arthritic change. Poor posture, increased weight, and/or misalignment of the spine or lower extremities each increase the mechanical stress placed upon a patient's joints. Short leg syndrome is especially stressful to lower extremity joints and it has been associated with increased incidence of hip osteoarthritis on the long leg side. It has also been implicated in temporomandibular joint dysfunction with subsequent arthritic change. Lack of joint motion as will occur with somatic dysfunction, encourages degeneration and fibrosis. It has been shown that passive range of motion can aid in cartilage regeneration. Like somatic dysfunction, arthritic change is usually manifested first in the minor motions of a joint.

Arthritic patients and many of the patients that have been improperly labeled as having "arthritis" have a great deal of myofascial somatic dysfunction. Travell and Simons report that clinically there is a high incidence of myofascial triggerpoints and tenderpoints in patients with joint problems. They have demonstrated that pain and tenderness in the joints of these "arthritic" patients often improve or disappear if the adjacent triggerpoints are treated. Treatment of myofascial somatic dysfunction, including triggerpoint treatment, frequently restores significant range-of-motion (ROM) to these joints. According to Travell this even seems to benefit joints that have appeared to have been ankylosed for years. Signs and symptoms including inflammation, effusion, soft tissue swelling and synovial crepitus frequently disappear.

There is a strong association between the somatic and the psychoemotional levels of patients who have myofascial triggerpoints. Surveys suggest that as many as 10% of these patients seek psychiatric care or think that they should. Many psychic effects commonly seen in rheumatologic patients (including depression and self-centeredness) have been reported to subside with treatment of myofascial somatic dysfunction.

LYMPHATICS:

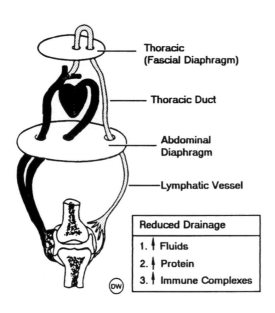

Thoracic
(Fascial Diaphragm)

Thoracic Duct

Abdominal
Diaphragm

Lymphatic Vessel

Reduced Drainage		
1. ↑ Fluids		
2. ↑ Protein		
3. ↑ Immune Complexes		

The effects of the sympathetic nervous system upon local circulation and the diffusion, nutrition and removal of waste products (including immune complexes) from a rheumatic joint have already been presented. (See page 160.) The lymphatics, however, are vital to the circulatory link and are particularly important in moving the immune complexes out of the area before they can cause damage to the joint. Manipulative treatment to enhance lymphatic homeostasis moves waste products out of the joint area thereby reducing diffusion gradients. This treatment begins with opening drainage pathways and is an integral part of rational osteopathic care.

Tendon sheaths are rich in lymphatic vessels and therefore lymphatic treatment should be utilized in tenosynovitis. Failure to reduce or relieve lymphatic congestion and the protein contained in the edematous fluid promotes fibrosis and thickening of the tissues. This, in turn, reduces ROM, encourages the formation of contractures around joints and subsequently further compromises lymphatic drainage.

It is known that immune reactions involving local synovial cells produce by-products which are associated with joint destruction proportional to their concentrations in the synovial fluid. In some severe cases, lymphoplasmaphoresis has been effectively used to promote diffusion gradients which are able to pull immune complexes out of the synovium. Expensive and dangerous surgical thoracic duct drainage has been found to be beneficial in some patients with systemic lupus erythematosus (SLE), myasthenia gravis, glomerulitis and rheumatoid arthritis.

PARASYMPATHETICS:

The parasympathetics play essentially no direct role in the musculoskeletal symptomatology of the arthritic patient; but because the body is a unit and rheumatologic disorders have chronic, systemic effects, consideration for improving the function of the parasympathetic nervous system in rheumatic patients is important because of its support of the visceral functions of the body.

OTHER FACTORS:

Patients with chronic arthritis become toxic, either from disease, their chronic use of medications, and/or from impaired excretion/metabolism. The physician managing patients with rheumatologic conditions must remain alert for side effects of medications or organ dysfunctions resulting from this toxicity. Total management of any chronic disease involves eliminating all foci of infection and visceral disease, supporting the patient's organs of detoxification and elimination, and supporting the known mechanisms of body homeostasis.

III. TREATMENT OF PATIENTS WITH RHEUMATOLOGIC DISORDERS

In order to address the rheumatologic patient's physical and psychologic needs, a rational treatment protocol must demonstrate the physician's understanding of the pathophysiology outlined above. General treatment goals include the following:

> o .. educate the patient regarding their disease process and the patient's own responsibilities in carrying out programs designed to maintain maximal function
> o .. provide psychologic support
> o .. alleviate pain and the pain-spasm-pain cycle

o .. decrease inflammation
o .. improve joint nutrition
o .. enhance removal of synovial waste products
o .. maintain and/or increase joint function
o .. decrease mechanical strain on affected joints
o .. correct existing deformity and prevent further deformity

OSTEOPATHIC MANIPULATIVE TECHNIQUES:

Recognizing the multisystem involvement of many of the rheumatologic disorders, assessment and treatment design in each of the involved systems are warranted. Soft tissue techniques address periarticular tissues and osteopathic manipulative treatments (OMT) reduce hypersympathetic activity and improve blood flow to the region. OMT directed toward removal of segmental facilitation also helps alleviate pain and pain perception. Tender and inflamed joints often respond best to indirect stacking or fascial unwinding manipulations, especially when prior structural changes may have roughened and modified joint surfaces. High velocity, low amplitude techniques (HVLA) are contraindicated in the cervical region of patients with severe rheumatoid arthritis because the high incidence of weakened cruciate ligaments is associated with potential pathologic subluxations.

In patients with inflammatory rheumatic disease, OMT may cause a transitory increase in joint pain; if this pain lasts more than 1-2 hours then either the choice of activation for the manipulative technique was incorrect or the dosage may have been excessive for that patient. A more general aching in the soft tissues may occur even with the most gentle activating forces (indirect). If this general ache lasts more than 24 hours it usually indicates that the physician attempted to produce more changes than the patient's body was capable of handling in a single visit and at that point in time. When this occurs, the OMT dosage and type should be evaluated and adjusted on the next visit.

After opening lymphatic drainage pathways and maximizing the patient's own respiratory pump, gentle joint pump techniques have been shown to be especially beneficial in granting pain relief. Posterior axillary fold technique (page 230) for patients with upper extremity congestion is particularly helpful. The value of intermittent non-weight-bearing compression of joint surfaces has been found to improve local nutrition and create beneficial histologic change in rheumatologic joints. The mechanisms active in this finding may explain the clinical results seen following this type of osteopathic manipulative treatment. It is not uncommon for morning stiffness, a hallmark sign in rheumatoid arthritis, to completely disappear after manipulative treatment is instituted and reasonably provided as part of the maintenance management program. Proper respiration and exercises directed toward maximizing respiratory abilities are also helpful in maintaining the lymphatic goals of treatment.

A variety of techniques including compression, Fluori-Methane^R spray and stretch, counterstrain positioning and injection have been shown to be beneficial in removing myofascial triggerpoints. It should be noted that the most common underlying or perpetuating factor associated with myofascial dysfunction is a postural disorder. For this reason and because postural problems directly and biomechanically stress the joints, postural analysis and treatment is often necessary before any other conservative treatment program for rheumatologic disease becomes effective. Postural correction may necessitate a shoe lift, Levitor^R orthotic device, or an orthotic shoe. Conservative treatment also includes patient education, osteopathic manipulative treatments, NSAIDs and/or other medications, exercise, and modifications of activities-of-daily-living (ADL).

Manipulative treatment of somatic dysfunction in the cranial region is frequently employed because of its possible role in affecting the pituitary gland's influence on the adrenal function, the essential steroidal hormones secreted by the adrenal cortex, and the pure sympathetic activity effect on the adrenal medulla. It is postulated that manipulation of somatic dysfunctions in the lower thoracic area also helps normalize hormonal levels through direct influence on adrenal function.

A physician who understands viscerosomatic reflexes and closely monitors the musculoskeletal system with palpatory examination has a substantial non-invasive advantage in the discovery of clues to visceral dysfunction. In the arthritic patient, musculoskeletal clues may be initiated by immune-complex deposition, toxicity from the medications used to treat chronic disease, or from mechanical change. If discovered at a dysfunctional level, steps can often be taken to prevent structural change. This connection is readily demonstrated when monitoring Chapman's reflex points, the celiac ganglion and the mid-thoracic paraspinal tissues in a patient taking NSAIDs. Early dysfunctional gastrointestinal signs warrant immediate intervention because structural changes in the form of gastritis and/or ulceration are common side effects of medical treatment for arthritis. Sometimes side effects warrant withdrawing certain medications from an otherwise successful medical treatment program. The finding of a previously absent musculoskeletal somatic dysfunction suspected of being viscerosomatic in nature, should prompt the physician to ask about new stressors as well as to review current medications. Often correcting the somatic dysfunction and then re-educating the patient to take their NSAIDs with food or discussing methods of stress management are adequate to reverse these early changes.

Treatment should be directed toward removal of factors contributing to spinal cord segmental facilitation and also toward maximizing function in target organs or in those organs important in the excretion of the toxins (liver, kidney, and bowel). It is known that the liver plays an important role in the clearance of soluble immune-complexes from the circulation and may play an important role in preventing immune-complexes from being deposited in vessel walls elsewhere in the body. Liver pump and CV4 techniques are frequently utilized to aid the body in general detoxification.

OTHER MANAGEMENT CONCERNS:

Some exercises are designed to maintain flexibility and others are designed to strengthen muscles where ligamentous support structures are inadequate. Walking programs as well as "aqua-cize" (water exercise) have both been shown to be beneficial to patients with rheumatoid arthritis.

The role of a specific dietary recommendation is nebulous at this time although some general recommendations are pertinent. Certainly weight control in obese patients is important in order to reduce biomechanical strain on joint structures. Patients with osteoarthritis are often over-weight while patients with rheumatoid arthritis are often under-nourished and warrant proper dietary education for general health reasons. While most texts state that diet is ineffective in managing arthritics, some patients are convinced that they experience arthritic flares with intake of certain foods such as sugar, citrus fruit, milk, fermented beverages, sodium benzoate, white flour, coffee and tea. Some physicians claim that there is a link between "food allergies" and arthritis. Some studies suggest that linoleic acid may be beneficial. Physicians can legitimately recommend a healthy diet as being appropriate for the patient regardless of any coexisting rheumatologic condition.

In patients with osteoporosis, bone mass is first lost in the anterior portion of the thoracic vertebrae making this area particularly susceptible to compression fractures. A loss of 30% of the bone mass is required before osteoporosis will be evident on x-rays. It is prudent to avoid high velocity, low amplitude treatments (HVLA) whenever osteoporosis is suspected. It is also best to substitute another technique that will accomplish the desired goal for any technique which places significant forward bending into the thoracic spine.

Patients with osteoarthritic changes may develop bony encroachment of the neural foramena in the cervical or lumbar regions. Backward bending or sidebending to the symptomatic side may increase the encroachment. Treatment goals include reducing excessive lordotic cervical and lumbar postural curves, promoting venous and lymphatic drainage in the area of the intervertebral area, and avoiding positioning which might aggravate the neural symptomatology.

Structural intervention is often necessary in patients with rheumatoid arthritis. In patients with significant joint effusion, drainage may prevent stretch of existing support structures and provide symptomatic relief for that patient.

Surgical intervention for structural joint deformities is often helpful in maintaining the patient's functional capabilities. The expertise of the rheumatologist and/or orthopedist and a team approach to the patient's needs can be extremely beneficial.

In patients with primary fibromyalgia syndrome who were already medicated with appropriate doses of Flexeril or amytryptaline, counterstrain OMT to tender points and systemic OMT to support homeostasis both improved subjective quality of life while reducing pain levels, but only the systemic OMT protocol was capable of reducing the number of tender points. After systemic OMT, 25% of patients in a KCOM study no longer fit the criteria for primary fibromyalgia established by the American College of Rheumatology.[*]

IV. SUMMARY: SUGGESTIONS FOR TREATMENT DESIGN

PATHOPHYSIOLOGY	OSTEOPATHIC CONSIDERATION
Arthritis <--> Somatic Dysfunction	1. Passive ROM 2. Correct Posture and Alignment 3. Fascial Indirect OMT 4. Joint Pumps
Toxic	1. Lymphatic Drainage 2. Liver and GB Pumps 3. CV4
Poor Cartilage Nutrition	1. Soft Tissue Periarticular Treatment 2. Indirect Stacking OMT 3. Joint Pumps
ANS Involvement	1. Treat Facilitated Segments 2. Decrease S/V and V/S Input 3. Rib Raising 4. Surg. or Rx Sympathetic Blockade if Severe
Inflammation	1. Anti-Inflammatory Rx 2. Anti-Rheumatic Rx in Severe Cases 3. Jnt. Pump and Lymphatic Protocols 4. Use non-traumatic OMT

RHEUMATOLOGIC BIBLIOGRAPHY:

*Lo KS, Kuchera ML, Preston SC, Jackson RW: Osteopathic manipulative treatment in fibromyalgia syndrome. JAOA 92(9):1177, Sept 1992. (JAOA article in review)

Stiles E: Osteopathic approach to rheumatoid arthritis. Osteopathic Medicine Aug 1977: 75-83.

Simkin PA: Synovial permeability in rheumatoid arthritis. Arthritis and Rheumatism 1979; 22 (7): 689-96.

Rothschild and Masi: Pathogenesis of rheumatoid arthritis: A vascular hypothesis. Seminars in Arthritis and Rheumatism 1982; 12 (1): 11-31.

Palmoski and Brandt: Aspirin aggravates the degeneration of canine joint cartilage caused by immobilization. Arthritis and Rheumatism 1982; 25 (11).

Wallace DJ et al: Plasmaphoresis and lymphoplasmophoresis in the management of rheumatoid arthritis. Arthritis and Rheumatism 1979; 22 (7): 703-10.

Cercere F et al: Evidence for the local production and utilization of immune reactants in rheumatoid arthritis. Arthritis and Rheumatism 1982; 25 (11): 1307-15.

Williams RC: Immunopathology of rheumatoid arthritis. Hospital Practice Feb 1978: 53-60.

Conditions of vessel wall deposition of immune complexes in immunologically induced vascular diseases, in Deicher and Shulz (ed) Arthritis--Models and Mechanism. Springer-Verlag, 1981.

Cochrane W et al: Absorptive functions of the synovial membrane. Ann Rheum Dis 1965; 24 (2): 2-15.

Levick JF: Contributions of the lymphatic and microvascular systems to fluid absorption from the synovial cavity of the rabbit knee. J Physio 1980; 306: 445-461.

Weissmann G: Mediators of tissue damage in rheumatoid arthritis: Phagocytes as secretory organs of rheumatoid inflammation. Triangle 1979; 18 (2/3): 45-52.

Enneking and Horowitz: The intra-articular effects of immobilization on human knee. Journal of Bone and Joint Surgery 1972; 54A: 973-85

Chrisman OD et al: The protective effect of aspirin against degeneration of human articular cartilage. Clinical Orthopaedics and Related Research 1972; 84: 193-196.

Mills and Sturrock: Clinical associations between arthritis and liver disease. Annals of the Rheumatic Diseases 1982; 41: 295-307.

INDEX OF APPENDIX

NOTES:

OSTEOPATHIC CONSIDERATIONS IN THE PEDIATRIC PATIENT

The modern general practice of pediatrics contains a large amount of preventive medicine. It offers the physician the opportunity to examine and begin a program for a patient that is healthy; usually the mother brings her well baby to you so that you can recommend and instruct her on measures (including nutrition, immunizations, and structural screening) that will optimize the health of this newborn infant (birth to age 2 years) or child (2 years old to puberty). Diagnosis and manipulative treatment programs for infants or children are different from those for adults; in a large part this diversity is due to certain anatomical and functional characteristics peculiar to the pediatric patient.

I. THE MUSCULOSKELETAL SYSTEM:

Though it is often said that the spine of the newborn is regionally flexed like a large C-curve, the lumbosacral angle actually begins to form as early as the fourth month of gestation age. The cervical curve has already begun to appear at birth and will increase with the efforts of the infant to raise the head and hold it erect. Activities like raising from the floor and crawling exercises develop the erector spinae muscles and begin to coordinate patterns of interaction between the nervous and musculoskeletal systems. The lumbar curve, however, does not appear until upright weight bearing is assumed. Its normal backward bending curvature gives spring to the spine and support of the pelvis, which then becomes the anchor for the hip extensors and rotators. Postural curves develop with weight bearing during childhood and postural abnormalities such as scoliosis can progress rapidly during growth spurts. Proper screening of posture should detect all scoliosis greater than 10 degrees;[1] scolioses measuring more than 20 degrees should have the benefit of a specialist's consultation. Secondary scoliosis can result from postural compensation for short leg syndrome, congenital spinal asymmetries, or even cranial somatic dysfunction which unlevels the eyes.

The musculoskeletal system of the infant and child is still developing. Most of the bones are cartilaginous to begin with and articulations between them are very elastic and resilient. Fryette's motion characteristics do not apply to the infant. Spinal motion patterns are nonspecific and restricted motion is usually due to local muscle contraction or fascial pull and not bony joint somatic dysfunction. The pediatric patient is surprisingly easy to treat. Although the child thinks that the physician is playing a game with them, treatment is not just haphazard but designed to move restricted joints and tissues through their ranges of motion. Dysfunctions "work themselves out;" it is seldom necessary to use thrusting type manipulation. Productive treatment time is very short with actual completion accomplished in about 2-3 minutes. Soreness as a reaction to treatment is rare.

II. THE IMMUNE SYSTEM:

Since the immune system is just developing, its lymphatic tissues take every opportunity to respond to an antigen; lymphadenopathy is often pronounced even with minor infections. Infectious diseases are common in children. In adults, viral adenopathy usually only involves the posterior cervical nodes. In children, viral lymphadenopathy can either involve anterior or posterior cervical lymphatic chains and usually results in an immune response that includes formation of large, thickened, tender, congested lymph nodes and overlaying skin that is moist, slick and hot. Anterior lymphadenopathy is often produced by bacterial infection and these nodes are usually shotty, coarse, grainy and are acutely tender to palpation.

It is clinically observed that infants and children respond rapidly to osteopathic manipulative treatment. Sometimes their temperature will increase a degree or two for a very short time after the treatment, then the fever will lyse and the temperature will drop to near normal. Parents should be told that this will happen. Children and infants get sick quickly but they also respond quickly to proper treatment and support of homeostatic mechanisms.

III. THE NERVOUS SYSTEM:

In the newborn, cranial somatic dysfunction from *in utero* forces or birth trauma may result and should be evaluated during the initial physical examination. Any obvious plagiocephaly or palpable cranial somatic dysfunction should be treated as soon as possible because both have been associated with pediatric otitis media,[2] attention deficit and learning disorders,[3] as well as colic, strabismus, suckling disorders, and a host of other symptoms associated with cranial nerve dysfunction. Dysfunction or injury to the nervous system is the most common serious consequence of a difficult birth and cranial OMT is ideally employed as early as possible to assist in structural-functional relationships. The pediatric history should always consider a narrative of the birth and perinatal period.

Neural connections are still developing so infants and children often react erratically, rapidly and very unpredictably to disease processes. With an infection, a newborn often reacts with decreased temperature and, often, bradycardia. In some newborns, the only symptoms of a severe infection may be eating poorly, regurgitating, becoming less active or more irritable or shaky. On the other hand, children (age two to puberty) may get very high temperatures with mild infections, or near normal temperatures with serious infections. Infants and children are also developing emotionally and socially. See page 179 for a graphic representation depicting some of this growth.

IV. OVERVIEW OF THE PEDIATRIC EXAMINATION:

At first, infants and young children may be frightened, because the physician is both a stranger and looks so big, tall, and threatening. Kneeling or sitting on a stool may help reduce their fears by making the physician more "their" size. It helps to appear happy and to always be kind and honest with these little patients. Some physicians do not wear a white coat because in the mind of the child, this may trigger some previous unfortunate, uncomfortable or frightening incident.

The first prerequisite to successful clinical encounters with children is to gain their confidence. It is essential that the physician knows the child's name and repeats it during questioning and conversation. The mother can promote security and safety by sitting close or holding the child on her lap during the examination; at other times, there are occasions when it is best to have the parent in the room, i.e. an overbearing parent or for an older child with a personal need for non-judgmental advice or direction. After greeting the mother and the patient, the very young child is best "ignored" while the history is taken by questioning the mother, with only apparent casual glances given to the child. He often doesn't understand the questions and, even if old enough to talk, the answers cannot be entirely believed, especially if not supported by physical and laboratory data. An adult often complains of pain and disability while a child notices inconveniences to playtime activity. The physician must deal more with objective signs as well as with the parent's anxieties about the child's problem. It helps to occasionally touch the infant on the foot, or briefly use some small talk during history taking. Avoid looking directly into the young child's eyes because this will usually produce a definite and immediate withdrawal response and often sets the tone for the rest of the pediatric patient/physician encounter.

During the early part of this visit, the physician often tries not to reveal a primary interest in the young child; in fact, it is best for the physician to obtain as much information as possible while taking the history from the parent and from casually observing the child's stance, activity level, and responses before beginning to directly examine the patient. Usually by the time the history is taken from the parent or primary care-giver and even though the physician has seemed to be uninterested in the infant or child, with observation and casual palpation metatarsal varus and tibial torsion have been evaluated. Sometime during this early encounter it is possible to see that the child is able to move the leg quickly and do so without pain.

While talking with the mother it is often possible to casually put a warm stethoscope on the chest of the infant or child and pretend not to know the stethoscope is there. He will look at the stethoscope, then at the physician (who is looking at and talking to the mother), then at the stethoscope again; he really is confused as to whether the physician is really doing anything to him or not. Before the child figures out that the physician is gathering information about the heart and lungs, the data has been obtained and no crying interferes with this important evaluation.

Be sure that the head of the stethoscope is warmed. A rubber-rimmed stethoscope bell will be less cold to the infant. Even a warm stethoscope or a stethoscope with a rubber ring around it apparently can feel cool and startle a child enough to make them cry. This suggested technique may improve chances of obtaining good auscultatory data from an infant and will usually keep him from crying: The physician's fingers are placed on the chest in about the position at which the stethoscope is to be placed; the infant or child does not seem to mind the touch of the hand, so the hand is placed on the chest with the fingers in the areas where the heart and/or lungs are to be auscultated. Then, one finger at a time is lifted and immediately replaced by the head of the stethoscope on the chest   The infant is usually unable to tell when the finger is lifted and replaced by the stethoscope, so remains relaxed and doesn't cry. A quiet infant or child improves the accuracy of auscultation.

Until a friendship has developed with you as the physician, never stare the young child or infant eye to eye. It is very threatening to them and they will try to get away as soon as the physician's eyes focus on theirs. It is necessary for the physician to gain their confidence before they permit eye contact. How this is accomplished depends upon the child's age and that undefinable "something" that is present between the physician and each of the young patients. After the child has become more accustomed to the physician, the cervical lymph glands can be evaluated by palpation. This can be performed effectively in a short period of time. Mobility of the hyoid and the anterior cervical fascias can be assessed at the same time. The abdomen is gently squeezed several times, looking for evidence of tenderness or masses. The ophthalmoscope is set at plus 8 diopters and at a distance of about 1 1/2 or 2 feet from the eye the light is flashed ("peek-a-boo") in the child's eyes looking for a red reflex.

The ears are then examined. It is safer and more information is quickly gathered using the biggest ear speculum in the diagnostic kit, even for the newborn infant. Remember to pull the ear down and back to open the external canal in an infant or young child. A single position of the speculum should visualize the entire tympanic membrane. Saying "peek-a-boo" makes the infant or young child think it's a game and he may hold very still. Examine the nose using the same large ear speculum. The diagnostic handle (light) must be held in such a way that the physician has good control during the examination so that any sudden, unexpected motion of the child is followed instantly by the otoscopic or auroscopic speculum to avoid scratch or contact damage of the canal, drum, or mucosa. Though it is not a scientific word, "yuck" often makes the young child laugh and present the other ear, nostril, or mouth to see if he can get the same response from the physician.

Some otoscopic diagnostic heads have a place to hold a tongue blade, but often these don't direct the light to the right place. Frequently in the infant, the light shines between their eyes instead of in the mouth. A special diagnostic head used only for holding the tongue blade and directing the light directly along the blade and into the mouth, is very helpful. If this special holder is not a part of your equipment, a bright penlight, held and operated on the tongue blade may be used. It allows the physician to control the light source and the tongue blade with one hand and have the other hand free to control the patient's head. If possible, have the child open the mouth wide and "pant like a puppy dog." The tongue will automatically pull down, the soft palate will rise and it becomes fairly easy to obtain a good view of the throat even without using the tongue blade. Tongue blades tend to frighten children.

Again, it is helpful to make infants and young children think you are playing with them. Sometimes the physician can hold the light up above the patient's head. When the child looks up at the light the mouth tends to open. Bring the tongue blade down and touch the mouth saying, "oops". When the child smiles or laughs, carefully but quickly slip the tongue blade over the tongue and look into the throat. A single gag, with you ready to quickly observe the view of the entire pharynx, often all the way to the epiglottis, is all that is usually required. Children seem to understand the words, "all done, " even at an early age; they often won't even cry. At that point turn away telling the child how good he/she was.

If the pediatric patient can stand, have him do so and assess his posture. Then have him bend over to touch his toes and look for a rib hump due to rotoscoliosis. If present, have the patient swing his trunk off to the right and left while still forward bent. The functional component of the rotoscoliotic curve will reduce.

Infants and children don't usually like to lie down in a physician's office. If you need to lay the infant down for some part of the examination such as Ortalani's test for a congenital hip disorder, do that procedure last, if at all possible. Often, once you lay the infant or child down, any friendship that has been established is lost.

This section does not describe an entire examination but offers an approach which considers the mind and spirit of the young child while beginning to examine the body. These suggestions tend to work most, but not all, of the time. Occasionally, there is a child who just won't cooperate. In this case, after taking the history and making a reasonable attempt to become friends, the exam must proceed in a calm, firm but gentle fashion using the humane

175

restraints of the mother and/or nurse, and a calm reassuring voice of the physician.

V. TREATMENT OF THE PEDIATRIC PATIENT:

Like osteopathic treatment of any patient, osteopathic manipulative treatment of a pediatric patient is based upon the application of principles and not upon formulae or techniques. Treating infants and children is often easy because they rarely have fibrosis and or chronic fixations; don't overtreat. Keep it simple and make it fun. Manipulative treatment is administered to the pediatric patient according to whether they are "pre-school" or "school age". Pre-school children only require articular mobilization and soft tissue. School-age children may require modified adult procedures.

Don't treat directly over infected lymphatic nodes; instead, treat around them and support the body systems that help the infant fight infection and recover from it effects. This means rib raising to reduce sympathetic hyperactivity while moving fluids and fascial techniques to dome the diaphragm and start the lymphatic pumps. Newborns and infants can be treated by placing them on the physician's thigh or by placing them in a lateral recumbent position of the table (your knee on the table in front of them) and administering soft tissue to the paraspinal tissues. The physician can also pick the child up and treat while walking around. The newborn can also be held against the chest and treated. A physician who has children can becomed experienced by treating his/her own children.

Insuring that the child gets solid foods during the time of high fever and anorexia is not as important as being sure that the child gets plenty of fluids. Children normally have a larger percentage of fluids in their bodies; many times a child or infant must be admitted to a hospital because of dehydration and not because of the disease process. So increase fluids, decongest peripheral tissues and return sequestered interstitial fluid back into the circulation by using lymphatic and fascial techniques."

Lymphatic pumps can be made fun for the child--"play with them". When the infant gets a little fussy or tries to get away from a rhythmic chest pump, suddenly stop and say, "Do you want more?" While they are trying to figure out why they should want more, start it again; when he fusses again, you say the same thing. Usually by the time he figures out that it's not really a game, the treatment is over; "all done." Another approach to "treatment" is to grasp feet and legs, lift their buttocks and their lower 2/3 of the body off the table, then jiggle the lower extremities gently. Flex one leg and then the other onto the chest, pushing each one gently and then extend the legs again. The child may be turned over by using the legs and then the physician may "play wheelbarrow" with them. This apparent play clinically promotes a type of lymph pump, fluid drainage, and movement of the body tissues. The mother can continue this "play-type" mobilization at home.

Remember, high velocity activation of osteopathic manipulative techniques is usually not required in infants and young children and because epiphyseal plates are still open, may not be the best choice of technique in this age group. Soft tissue treatment and articulatory methods of treatment are very effective and make it fun for the child. Again, do not over-treat. There is the "tick-tock method" of treatment, in which the physician holds the chest of the child under the arms and rocks him back and forth, from right to left, mobilizing the spine and other tissues. The fascias of the thoracic inlet and the diaphragmatic area should be treated. If the infant is getting an exanthema or prodromal of an infectious disease, treatment clinically results in less rash, less fever and a decrease in the severity of the disease. Pediatric patients benefit from osteopathic diagnosis and manipulative treatment and both should be integrated into pediatric care.

Inform the parents that commonly after manipulative treatment, the temperature will briefly go up in a pediatric patient before coming down. Also educate them that fever is not necessarily bad. Increased temperature is one of the body's ways of mobilizing defenses against an infection. Viruses multiply best at temperatures slightly below normal. Fever hinders viral replication and is a way of increasing circulation and getting the immune substances to the infected areas, helping the infant's own homeostatic mechanisms. It increases metabolism and circulation and creates an environment poorly tolerated by microorganisms.

Fever that is too high may cause convulsions and the threshold for convulsions from fever varies from child to child; therefore, its level must be controlled. If there is a febrile seizure history, then the physician must be more cautious in instructing the parents in maintaining temperature control in the infant or child. Aspirin may be associated with development of Reyes' Syndrome and therefore it is not as good an antipyretic choice as acetaminophen. As a rule of thumb, a fever under 101°F doesn't need to be treated. Above 102°F a dose of acetaminophen (1 grain per age of life) could be given.

A physician knows that his/her management of a child has been successful if a mother brings in one of her children and says, "Johnny cried because he wanted to come in and see his doctor too." If you desire to read more on examination of the child, read "How to examine a baby or a small child and how to keep your cool" written by retired pediatrician, Robert Mercer, M.D.[4] You can feel the joy he had in being able to care for infants and children. Dr. Mercer says, "The real reward of a successful examination is when the small person climbs up on your lap for further friendly play; then you know for sure that you have done a good job and established a new friendship in the process." When the child likes "the doctor," a satisfying patient encounter becomes even more enjoyable.

REFERENCES:

1. Kuchera WA, Kuchera ML: <u>Osteopathic Principles in Practice</u>. 2nd edition. KCOM Press, Kirksville MO, 1992, p 352.
2. Degenhardt BD, Kuchera ML: The prevalence of cranial dysfunction in children with a history of otitis media from kindergarten to third grade. Mead-Johnson Fellowship Paper, 1993
3. Frymann V: Relation of disturbances of craniosacral mechanism to symptomatology of the newborn: Study of 1,250 infants. <u>JAOA</u> 65:1059-1075, 1966
4. Mercer RD: How to examine a baby or a small child and keep your cool. <u>Cleveland Clinic Quarterly</u> Fall 1983; 50: 255-261.

PEDIATRIC GROWTH (Adapted from Wessel)[1]

Hungry for companionship, staring is a baby's way of reaching out to others. Reaching for the closeness necessary for healthy development. The infant progresses from the ability to barely see to complex talents including coordination to seek, to remember, and to imitate.

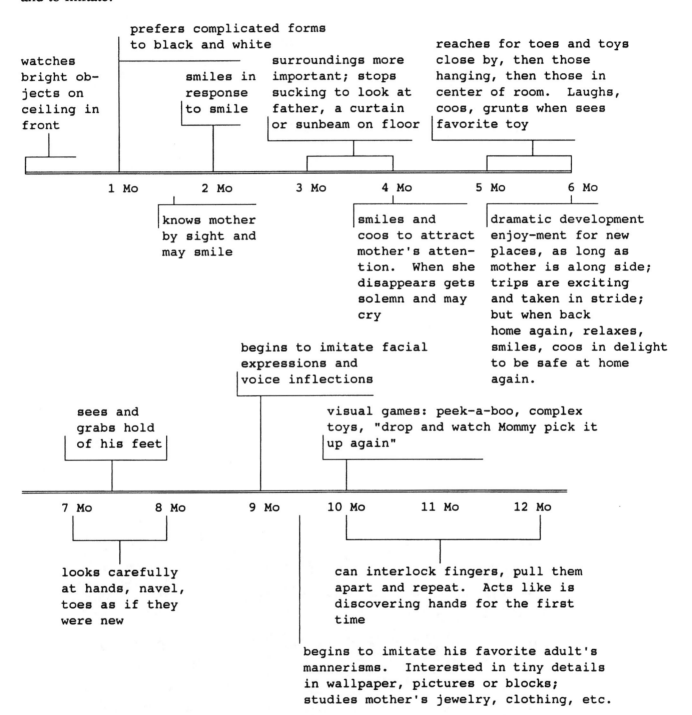

1. Wessel, MA; From A Baby's Point Of View: Associate Professor Of Pediatrics At Yale University.

179

Still-Hildreth Osteopathic Sanatorium

Macon, Missouri

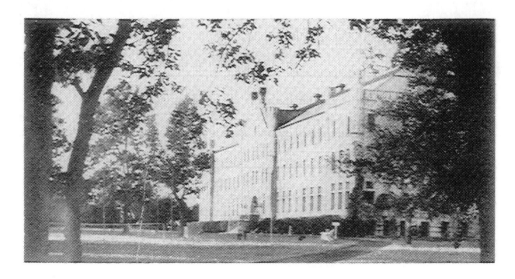

Dedicated to the Treatment and Care of Nervous
and Mental Patients

1914   1939

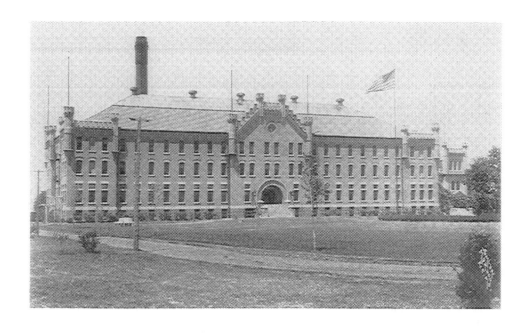

OSTEOPATHIC CONSIDERATIONS IN PSYCHIATRY
BIBLIOGRAPHY

Bradford, Spencer, G.; Role Of Osteopathic Manipulative Therapy In Emotional Disorders: A Physiologic Hypothesis; JAOA; Vol. 64; No. 7; Jan 1965: 64-73

Dunn, Floyd E.; Osteopathic Concepts In Psychiatry; JAOA; Vol. 49; No. 7; Mar 1950: 354-357

Espeland, Darryl, and Peters, Christian; OMT And Substance Abuse Rehabilitation; Osteopathic Annals; Vol. 13; Feb 1985: 26-30

Sackler, Arthur M.; Restricted Blood Flow In Brain Found In Some Schizophrenics; Medical Tribune; Jan 11, 1984

Woods, John M.; Woods, Rachel H.; A Physical Finding Related To Psychiatric Disorders; JAOA; Vol. 60; Aug 1961: 988-993

OSTEOPATHIC CONSIDERATIONS IN IMMUNOLOGY
BIBLIOGRAPHY:

Amalfitano, D.M.; The Osteopathic Thoracic-Lymphatic Pump: A Review of the Historical Literature; Journal of Osteopathic Medicine; Apr-May, 1987: 20-24

Gunderson TG, Gordon RM: A study of the influence of spinal lesions on the course of infections. JAOA 1932; 31: 390.

Measel, J.W.; The Effect of Lymphatic Pump in the Immune Response: I. Preliminary Studies in the Antibody Response to Pneumococcal Polysaccharide Assayed by Bacterial Agglutination and Passive Hemagglutination; JAOA; 82 (1): 28-31

Measel, J.W.; Introduction: Thoughts in Osteopathic Practice and Infectious Diseases; Osteopathic Annals; 10 (3); Mar 1982: 7-11

Measel, J.W., et. al,; The Effect of the Lymphatic Pump in the B and T Cells in Peripheral Blood; Osteopathic Annals; JAOA; 86 (9); Sep 1896: 608

Paul, R., et. al.; Interferon Levels in Human Subjects Throughout a 24-hour Period Following Thoracic Lymphatic Pump Manipulation; JAOA; 86 (2); Feb 1986: 92-95

Purse FM: Clinical evaluation of osteopathic manipulative therapy in measles. JAOA 1961; 61: 274.

Thorpe, R.; Osteopathic Manipulative Therapy for Infection; Osteopathic Annals; 8 (9); Sep 1980: 30-34

The proceedings of an International Conference on this subject will soon be available from the American Academy of Osteopathy. Conference co-chairpersons were Frank Willard, PhD and Michael Patterson, PhD.

HYPERSYMPATHETIC ACTIVITY ON SELECTED TISSUES
EXTRACTED FROM COLLECTED PAPERS OF I.M. KORR, PHD
1977-1989

> Sympathetic hyperactivity does not introduce any new qualities, only modifies the inherent functional properties of the target tissues.

SKELETAL MUSCLE:

o .. Augments contraction similar to inotropic effect on cardiac muscle, "Orbeli effect"
o .. Facilitates neuromuscular transmission
o .. Increases contracture formation after spinal cord trauma

PERIPHERAL SENSORY MECHANISM:

o .. Facilitation: increases rate of discharge and lowers threshold to fire (may reach zero so that fires without direct stimulation of receptor)
o .. Exaggeration of response: reports a greater intensity of stimulation than is actually occurring; increases or exaggerates the perception of pain
o .. The sensory mechanisms that have been demonstrated to respond in this manner include:

--muscle spindle   --tactile receptors
--taste receptors   --olfactory apparatus
--Pacinian corpuscles   --retina and cochlea
--carotid sinus chemoreceptors

CENTRAL NERVOUS SYSTEM:

o .. Strong influential connection between hypersympathetic activity in superior cervical ganglion and subcortical activity, especially on the ipsilateral side
o .. Primary influence is on the mechanisms responsible for generation of the background electrical activity, the rhythm assimilation reaction and the secondary components of the induced reaction to light
o .. Facilitating effects have been observed in the reticular formation, general brain, cerebellum and spinal cord

COLLATERAL CIRCULATION:

o .. There is a decrease in development of collateral circulation; sympathectomy increases the development of collateral circulation in areas of occlusion

o .. There is decreased mortality and morbidity in experimentally induced myocardial infarction when sympathetics are cut

ADIPOSE TISSUE:

o .. Sympathetics are requisite for lipolysis independently from blood flow (alpha for vasculature and beta for adipose tissue)

o .. Increases in glycogenolysis requires increased oxygen

ENDOCRINE SYSTEM:

o .. Sympathetic significantly influences the pineal gland and thereby influences other endocrine systems; this is especially related to sexual development and reproduction. Superior cervical ganglion influence on the pineal gland through synthesis of melatonin

BONE GROWTH:

o .. Reduces the growth of longitudinal bone

RETICULOENDOTHELIAL SYSTEM:

o .. Increases circulating reticulocytes and normoblasts

SOME SPECIFIC CLINICAL REACTIONS TO SYMPATHICOTONIA:

ARTERIOSCLEROSIS:

Sustained stimulation of sympathetics produce histologic features of arteriosclerosis and increases tendency towards thrombosis.

HYPERTENSION:

High activity of the peripheral sympathetic nervous system is felt to be an important contributing factor in some forms of arterial hypertension.

HEART:

Increased sympathetic activity increases oxygen demands which contribute to the extent and degree of cardiac ischemia and angina.

Sympathicotonia increases the extent of myocardial damage following an MI.

(Experiments with cats) Post-MI there is a higher discharge of sympathetic activity at T3 ramus communicans, termed a cardio-cardiac reflex, which plays and important role in increased rate of dysrhythmia and ventricular fibrillation. Sympathicotonia also lowers threshold to the development of ectopic foci in the heart. Adrenergic blockade protects the heart from these effects especially in the few hours post-MI and lowers the mortality rates.

Increased sympathetic impulses to the kidney is implicated in the retention of Na^+ and water in CHF patients.

PEDIATRICS:

Increased sympathetic activity has been implicated in the long Q-T interval associated with Sudden Infant Death Syndrome.

URETERAL CALCULI:

Ureteral calculi produce ipsilateral facilitation of sympathetic activity. Increased sympathetic activity is also implicated in poor ureteral transport of fluids, a factor in calculi formation. If calculi are present in the ureter, sympathetic hyperactivity decreases the peristalsis of the ureters which hinders removal of the calculus from the ureter.

Superimposed emotions associated with increased sympathetic responses may are found to reduce glomerular filtration rate (GFR).

THE SKELETAL SYSTEM:

Hypersympathetic activity retards bone growth. Sympatholytic treatment restores bone growth to a normal rate.

There is reduced rheumatoid and osteoarthritic disease in the extremities following sympathectomy.

THE EXTREMITIES:

Prolonged sympathetic activity in response to significant or relatively insignificant trauma results in "reflex sympathetic dystrophy", a syndrome including heightened pain, trophic changes, osteoporosis, connective tissue disease, and an extremity that is cool, sweaty, cyanotic, chronically edematous, and has thickened nails. Often these changes are responsive to sympathectomy.

LIVER:

Sympathetic bombardment releases fatty acids from the periphery and deposits them in the liver.

PANCREAS:

Sympathetic stimulation can convert a mild, nonlethal type of bile-induced pancreatitis into the necrotizing, hemorrhagic lethal form. This is probably secondary to vasoconstriction and slight ischemia of the pancreas.

OTHER AREAS OF HYPERSYMPATHETIC EFFECT:

Glaucoma, colitis, megacolon, peripheral vascular disease, postoperative paralytic ileus, Dupuytren's contracture, irritable bowel syndrome (IBS), pelvic congestion in women, etc.

AUTONOMIC NERVOUS SYSTEM INFLUENCE IN SELECTED AREAS		
STRUCTURE	SYMPATHETIC	PARASYMPATHETIC
Pupil	Dilation	Constriction
Ciliary Muscle	--------	Contraction
Lacrimal Gland	--------	Secretory
Mucous Glands (N-Th)	Inhibition	Secretory
Parotid Gland	Inhibition	Secretory
Submaxillary Gland	Inhibition	Secretory
Sublingual Gland	Inhibition	Secretory
Blood Vessels (Skin)	Vasoconstriction	--------
Pilomotor Muscles	Contraction	--------
Sweat Glands	Secretory	--------
Common Carotid Artery	Vasoconstriction	--------
Mucous Glands (phx-larx)	Vasoconstriction	Secretory
Thyroid Gland	Vasoconstriction	--------
Heart	Excitation	Inhibition
Bronchial Muscle	Relaxation	Contraction
Bronchial Glands	Inhibition	Secretory
Upper Body Vasculature	Vasoconstriction	--------
Stomach	Inhibition	Motor and Secretion
Liver	Glycogenolysis	Glycogen Synthesis
Spleen	Vasoconstriction	--------
Gallbladder and Ducts	Relaxation	Contraction
Pancreas	Inhibition	Secretory

AUTONOMIC NERVOUS SYSTEM INFLUENCE IN SELECTED AREAS (cont)		
STRUCTURE	**SYMPATHETIC**	**PARASYMPATHETIC**
Kidney	Vasoconstriction	--------
Adrenal Medulla	Adrenaline Secretion	--------
Intestinal Tract	Contraction	Relaxation
Rectal Sphincter	Contraction	Relaxation
Vesicle Sphincter	contraction	Relaxation
Vesicle Body	Relaxation	Constriction
Uterine Fundus	constriction	Relaxation
Uterine Cervix	Relaxation	Constriction
Male Reproductive Organs	Ejaculation	Erection
Ovary and Testes	Vasoconstriction	(unknown)

REFERRED PAIN: Generally, visceral afferent nerves from the viscera follow the same pathway as traveled by the sympathetic innervation of the organ. Impulses from visceral nerve endings arrive among the posterior horn cells as do impulses of somatic origin. Visceral referred pain will be noted in the somatic segment(s) which share the same dorsal horn lamina V of neurons. There may be superficial skin changes, reflex muscle spasm and vasomotor changes.

o .. Visceral referred pain may be gripping, cramping, aching, crushing, squeezing, tearing, stabbing or burning.
o .. It is usually poorly localized.
o .. Referred pain may have rhythmic occurrence to it.

From hollow viscus: greatest intensity in 20-30 sec, lasts 2 minutes, quickly subsides, and reoccurs again in minutes. From vascular areas: throbbing pain from inflammation and chemical mediators; it increases in severity and lasts an extended period of time.

o .. Usually associated with other symptoms of visceral disease.
o .. People with viscerogenic pain get no relief from rest; they find more comfort if moving, trying to find a position of comfort.
o .. See pages 79-82 for diagrammatic depiction of pain progression.

___

OSTEOPATHIC MANIPULATIVE TECHNIQUES

USE OF OSTEOPATHIC MANIPULATIVE TREATMENT IN SYSTEMIC DYSFUNCTION

Dysfunction and disease change the local and regional intercellular environments. An increase in interstitial tissue fluids is one of the results of this tissue dysfunction. Resulting congestion disturbs local and regional biochemical homeostasis. Disease and dysfunction also provoke receptors of visceral afferent and/or somatic sensory nerves which then flood their spinal cord areas with neural impulses. Afferent (sensory) impulses usually follow the same fascial pathways as the sympathetic nerves innervating the affected organ or organs. Occasionally, as from the alveoli of the lungs or from the cervix of the uterus, visceral afferents follow the pathways of the organ's parasympathetic supply. In either case, constant bombardment by visceral afferent impulses facilitates the spinal cord segments at their destination. This means a reduction in the threshold of the synapses in the neuronal pool of the dorsal horn in those regions of the spinal cord. Because there is "cross-talk" between these pools, palpable somatic changes result from visceral dysfunction and visceral dysfunction can also result from somatic dysfunction. Once facilitated cord segments are established, stress of any kind (physical, mental or emotional) will initiate an outburst of sympathetic impulses to their associated viscera even if that stress has no direct relationship to the low threshold segments.

Successful osteopathic manipulative treatment for patients with systemic dysfunction or disease has these common goals:

o .. Reduce the two main factors responsible for initiating or sustaining facilitated spinal cord segments, whether they be associated with somatic and/or visceral dysfunction.
o .. Support homeostatic mechanisms by reducing somatic and visceral factors that contribute to the maintenance of spinal cord facilitation. Reduction of cord facilitation enables the body to make more appropriate reflex responses to proprioceptive input.
o .. Support biomechanical mechanisms responsible for moving lymphatic fluids from the interstitial spaces back to the circulation and for removing metabolic by-products and medications from the intercellular environment. This aids fluid homeostasis throughout the body.
o .. Support the parasympathetic nervous system by treatment of fascial restrictions and somatic dysfunction in the regions of the sphenopalatine ganglion, the cranium, the OA or the sacrum. These treatments promote balance within the autonomic system and prepares the body to return toward a homeostatic level which is more physiologic for that patient.

o .. Support the body processes and mechanisms which allow the body to
metabolize and use the food that is taken into the body.
o .. Support the mental, spiritual and emotional needs of the patient.

It should be readily apparent why initial osteopathic manipulative treatment is often directed toward reducing facilitation and promoting a more appropriate sympathetic response. The treatment program will usually progress toward support of the body's lymphatic system; and finally, toward effecting parasympathetic balance. Osteopathic manipulative management is specific for each patient, providing treatment indicated by the history of that patient, the known natural history of the disease process, and the palpatory findings on examination of the patient. There are a variety of manipulative techniques that can be used to affect somatic dysfunction, the autonomic nervous system, and the lymphatics. It must be re-emphasized that the manipulative portion of a management program is unique for each patient and is planned according to each patient's individual needs.

A basic plan for the efficient use of the patient's neuromusculoskeletal system during the formulation of a differential diagnosis and treatment plan is very helpful. The following figure is a model for such a plan. It has been found to be clinically useful in effectively and efficiently formulating and executing supportive osteopathic manipulative treatment for a patient with systemic disease.

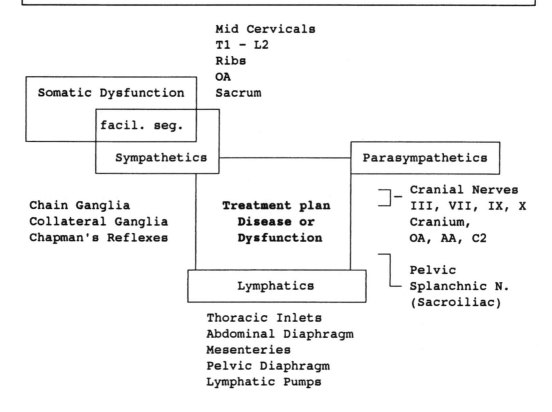

SYMPATHETIC AND PARASYMPATHETIC INNERVATION

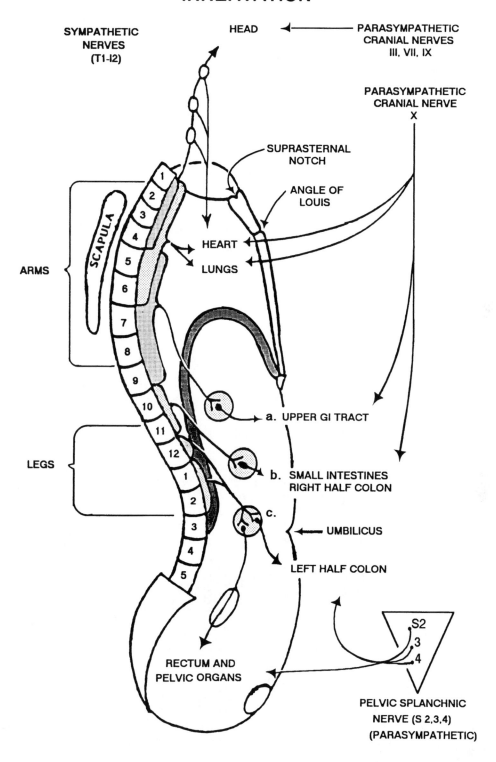

SYMPATHETIC
NERVES
(T1-I2)

HEAD

PARASYMPATHETIC
CRANIAL NERVES
III, VII, IX

PARASYMPATHETIC
CRANIAL NERVE
X

SUPRASTERNAL
NOTCH

ANGLE OF
LOUIS

SCAPULA

ARMS

HEART

LUNGS

a. UPPER GI TRACT

b. SMALL INTESTINES
RIGHT HALF COLON

LEGS

c.

UMBILICUS

LEFT HALF COLON

S2
3
4

RECTUM AND
PELVIC ORGANS

PELVIC SPLANCHNIC
NERVE (S 2,3,4)
(PARASYMPATHETIC)

COMPOSITE AUTONOMIC INNERVATION CHART

PARASYMPATHETIC INNERVATIONS

CRANIOSACRAL	VISCERA	THORACO-LUMBAR
CRANIAL III	– PUPILS	T1-4
CRANIAL VII	– LACRIMAL AND SALIVARY GLANDS	T1-4
CRANIAL VII	– SINUSES	T1-4
CRANIAL IX, X	– CAROTID BODY AND SINUS	T1-4
CRANIAL X VAGUS	– THYROID	T1-4
"	– TRACHEA/BRONCHI	T1-6
?	– MAMMARY GLANDS	T1-6
CRANIAL X VAGUS	– ESOPHAGUS LOWER 2/3	
"	– AORTA	
"	– HEART	T1-6
"	– LUNGS AND VISCERAL PLEURA	T1-6
"	– STOMACH	T5-9L
"	– DUODENUM	T5-9
"	– LIVER	
"	– GALL BLADDER AND DUCTS	T5R
"	– SPLEEN	T6R
"	– PANCREAS	T7L
"	– RIGHT COLON	T7R
?	– OVARY AND TESTES	T10-11
CRANIAL X VAGUS	– SMALL INTESTINES	T10-11
"	– KIDNEY	T10-11
"	– ENTIRE COLON	T10-L2
"	– APPENDIX	T12

SYMPATHETIC INNERVATIONS

REGIONAL AREAS	CORD LEVEL	SPLANCHNIC NERVES	COLLATERAL GANGLIA
HEAD AND NECK	T1-4		(CERV. GANGLIA)
HEART	T1-6		(CERV. GANGLIA)
LUNGS	T1-6		----
ENTIRE GI TRACT:	T5-L2		
UPPER GI TRACT	T5-9	GREATER SPLANCHNIC	CELIAC GANGLION
SM INT./RHT COLON	T10-11	LESSER SPLANCHNIC	SUP. MESENTERIC GANGLION
APPENDIX	T12	LEAST AND LUMBAR SPLANCHNIC	
LEFT COLON/PELVIS	T12-L2		INF. MESENTERIC GANGLION
ADRENAL	T10-11		
KIDNEY	T10-11		

Continued on next page

192

Continuation of autonomic innervation chart:

COMPOSITE AUTONOMIC INNERVATION CHART

PARASYMPATHETIC INNERVATIONS			SYMPATHETIC INNERVATIONS			
CRANIOSACRAL	VISCERA	THORACO-LUMBAR	REGIONAL AREAS	CORD LEVEL	SPLANCHNIC NERVES	COLLATERAL GANGLIA
PELV. SPLANCHNICS	LEFT COLON –	T12-L2				
(NONE)	ADRENAL	T10-11				
VAGUS	UPPER URETER –	T10-11	UPPER URETER	T10-11		
PELV. SPLANCHNICS	LOWER URETER –	T12-L1	LOWER URETER	T12-L1		
"	BLADDER (BODY) –	T12-L2	BLADDER	T12-L2		
"	BLADDER TRIGONE AND SPHINCTER –	T12-L2				
"	UTERINE BODY –	T12-L2				
"	PROSTATE –	T12-L2				
"	GENITAL CAVERNOUS TISSUES					
(NONE)	ARMS –	T2-8				
(NONE)	LEGS –	T11-L2				

* PELVIC SPLANCHNIC = S 2,3,4 (PARASYMPATHETIC)

193

In order to use this plan, it is necessary to be familiar with sympathetic and parasympathetic innervations for groups of organs. This is often where the plan fails, because a physician may have trouble remembering the autonomic innervations to organs. For this reason, sympathetic innervations of various viscera were reviewed in many anatomical and neurological texts where there seemed to be a wide and variable range of sympathetic innervation to any one organ. Common visceral innervations were then grouped so that they could be easily memorized while still maintaining their clinical relevance. The result was the composite chart of autonomic innervation on pages 192 and 193. This chart retains credible correlation with all of the different ranges of sympathetic innervation presented by various authors, but is also much easier to memorize. Recognize that intense visceral afferent activity from certain clinical situations may result in a spread of the facilitated cord segments up or down in the thoracolumbar spinal cord area and result in an increased range of palpable somatic paraspinal involvement initiated by that organ system dysfunction. It may even result in the expression of symptoms from other systems or organs that happen to be innervated by sympathetic fibers from adjacent cord segments.

II. TREATMENT SYMPATHETIC NERVOUS SYSTEM DYSFUNCTION:

A. TREATMENT GOALS AND GENERAL MANIPULATIVE TREATMENT PLAN:

Organs which are primarily or secondarily involved in dysfunction exhibit characteristic changes or symptomatology of sympathicotonia. Diagnosis and treatment can be directed to several anatomic-physiologic locations: The thoracolumbar paraspinal chain ganglia, the collateral sympathetic (preaortic and cervical) ganglia, through the facilitated spinal cord segments, or through specific reflex systems such as Chapman's and Travell's myofascial points. The spinal cord segments can be maintained in their facilitated state by being bombarded by visceral or somatic afferent fibers from visceral and/or somatic dysfunctions.

Set Goals: Because the sympathetic chain ganglia are anatomically located anterior to the rib heads, any dysfunction that directly or indirectly and "chronically" restricts fascia in this region may initiate and/or maintain excessive sympathetic outflow to their reference organs. It naturally follows that normal rib motion as well as reduced afferent input from paraspinal muscles or the viscera, will help to reduce segmental cord facilitation.

Abdominal collateral sympathetic ganglia are able to control local and perhaps some regional autonomic responses without reporting to the CNS. These ganglia are also in the pathway of the visceral afferents that relay impulses of GI or pelvic dysfunction to the CNS.

Animal studies have revealed evidence that early manipulation of somatic dysfunction might act as a form of preventive medicine. Summarizing some of his animal studies, Patterson[1] purports:

o .. Persistent musculoskeletal dysfunction affecting a certain spinal cord
        segment can affect the function of an internal organ related to that same
        spinal cord segment.
o .. Removal of the musculoskeletal irritation produced by dysfunction allows
        the related internal organ to return to its normal function.
o .. If the dysfunction of the musculoskeletal system remains long enough, it
        apparently "burns a memory pattern" within the central nervous system
        so that when the initial irritating musculoskeletal influence is removed,
        the original dysfunction not only continues but grows in severity.

B. RIB RAISING TECHNIQUES:

Ribs should also move well to permit painless, effortless breathing. The diaphragm is the extrinsic pump of the lymphatic system. Good diaphragmatic action is supported by treatment of specific rib somatic dysfunction and by rib raising techniques that increase the depth of respiration. Treatment of somatic dysfunction and the mechanical principles applied in "rib raising" techniques provoke maximum excursion of the rib cage, encourage maximum inhalation and the generation of more effective negative intrathoracic pressure. This increases lymphatic flow and also relaxes the patient. These techniques also help to re-establish range-of-motion and thereby reduce excessive afferent input to facilitated cord segments.

Rib raising is actually the primary manipulative method by which the osteopathic physician affects the hypersympathetic activity initiated by dysfunction or disease. Effective rib raising techniques lift and rotate the rib heads; they, in turn, pull on the fascias that are common to a rib head and its sympathetic chain ganglion. This initially "stimulates" reflex sympathetic responses in the related organs, an event which the physician usually wishes to reduce and prevent, especially as a long term circumstance. Reflex neurophysiologists explain that the sympathetic activation produced by rib raising is due to stimulation of fast and very fast efferent sympathetic fibers but that this response is fairly localized and short lived. They also report that rib raising techniques will additionally stimulate slow and very slow efferent sympathetic fibers in the same ganglia and these fibers reflex as high as the medullary centers. These latter reflexes are reported to be inhibitory to the sympathetic system and also are long acting.

It is important to reduce the sensitivity of the spinal areas demonstrating increased facilitation first, so that proprioceptor impulses produced by treatment of other areas will not produce firing of these segments with lowered thresholds. An optimal treatment protocol strives to maximize the body's own homeostatic ability to maintain rib motion -- thus, dysfunction of the thoracics, sternum, diaphragm (including lumbar attachments and cervicophrenic innervation), and cranial elements might be considered and be appropriately treated. If a physician applies the basic principles of rib raising treatment, a variety of techniques can be formulated for utilization in the management of patients who are in a variety of positions and who have a variety of medical conditions.

RIB RAISING FOR ACUTELY DEBILITATED PATIENTS: PATIENT SUPINE

o .. Purpose(s):

> o .. To decrease sympathetic facilitation
> o .. To increase respiratory efficiency and depth
> o .. To increase lymphatic return
> o .. To reduce general stress and discomfort

o .. The operator sits beside patient and inserts both hands under the patient contacting the angles of the ribs with the fingers of both hands.
o .. The operator must lift up (toward ceiling) sufficiently to move the rib and its rib head (sternum should also rise) and pull slightly lateral to the point of tissue resistance--ease of performing the lift is gained by using the dorsal surface of the MCP joints as a fulcrum against the bed or table.
o .. Additional lymphatic and/or respiratory benefits may possibly be gained by using the hands and/or finger pads to pressure the ribs towards inhalation (pump handle inhalation encouragement requires a caudal direction from the finger pads at the posterior aspect of the rib to bring the anterior portion superiorly; bucket handle rib motion requires a cephalad pull from the posterior contact). The sympathetic effect of rib raising as described is probably effective without any of this specially directed activity.
o .. When the tissues relax, the operator should slowly reposition his or her hands onto the next group of adjacent untreated rib angles and repeat the procedure. The other side of the rib cage is treated in the same manner until the entire rib cage has been treated.

RIB RAISING TECHNIQUE FOR LESS DEBILITATED PATIENTS: PATIENT SUPINE

o .. Purpose(s): Same as above.
o .. The operator stands at the head of the patient.
o .. The patient is supine and reaches up with both arms over head to encourage raising of the ribs and in some manner, affixes hands around the posterior aspect of the operator's waist or to a belt (or other material).
o .. The operator contacts the patient's rib angles by sliding the hands under each side of the chest cage (approaching the rib angles from the sides of the rib cage).
o .. The operator must lift up (toward ceiling) and lean backward sufficiently to move the ribs and their rib heads.
o .. As the operator lifts and leans backwards and downward, the pull through the patient's arms stretches the pectoral and latissimus dorsi muscles, encouraging the ribs into inhalation
o .. This lift from the head of the bed or table is repeated until the ribs move easily.

RIB RAISING FOR A SEATED PATIENT:

This is an especially helpful technique for patients that are uncomfortable or unable to lie down.

o .. Patient is seated with arms crossed, the shoulders are flexed and the head rested on the arms
o .. Operator stands at side of patient and supports the crossed arms with one upper extremity; the other hand is placed across the patient's thoracic spine contacting bilaterally as much of the rib as possible
o .. The patient is instructed to relax their back and allow their weight to fall forward onto the operator's supporting arm
o .. The operator lifts and allows the patient to transfer their weight farther forward onto the supporting arm; the other hand is used to create a fulcrum in the thoracic spine for backward bending
o .. The process above is applied to the entire rib cage as is comfortable to the patient

MUSCLES USED IN MUSCLE ENERGY RIB TECHNIQUES USED TO ELEVATE OR DEPRESS RIB SOMATIC DYSFUNCTIONS (SD):

Muscles used to elevate exhalation rib SD	
Scalenes	Ribs 1-2
Pectoralis Minor	Ribs 3,4,5 (6)
Serratus Anterior	Ribs 6,7,8,9,10
Latissimus Dorsi	Ribs 9,10,11,12
(Quadratus Lumborum)	Rib 12 (indirectly)
Intercostals	Forced inhalation

Muscles used to depress inhalation rib SD	
Quadratus Lumborum	Rib 12 (directly)
Intercostalis	Forced exhalation

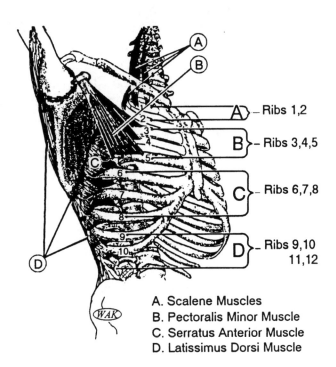

A – Ribs 1,2
B – Ribs 3,4,5
C – Ribs 6,7,8
D – Ribs 9,10 11,12

A. Scalene Muscles
B. Pectoralis Minor Muscle
C. Serratus Anterior Muscle
D. Latissimus Dorsi Muscle

THE ILEUS PREVENTION TREATMENT: ("RIB RAISING" AREAS WITHOUT RIBS)

Producing the effects of rib raising in these segments could not be performed through rib heads. The following describes an inhibition technique for the L1 to L2 spinal area, but the same technique can be used to treat the effects of hypersympathetic outflow in the thoracic area.

o .. The patient is supine and the physician is seated at the side of the patient.
o .. The physician passes both hands under the back the patient to a point where the finger tips are on one side and the thenar and hypothenar eminences are on the other side of the erector spinae mass (ESM).
o .. The hands are then closed, pulling the two erector spinae mass muscles toward each other between the fingers and the thenar/hypothenar eminences of the operator.
o .. This maneuver automatically lifts or backward bends the spinal region located above the hands. If the operator's hands were in an area of ribs, this backward bending would be enough to perform effective rib raising.

198

o .. The pressure on the operator's fingers and heel of the hands is equalized by altering the pressure on these structures, resulting in a slight rotation of the patient's body to the right or left.

o .. Further balance between the hands and the patient's back is adjusted by pushing or pulling one forearm away or toward the operator's body until the pressure on the two hands is about equal.

o .. When pressures are balanced, the hands remain gripping the ESM until there is a sense of relaxation (usually about 60-90 seconds).

o .. Re-gripping the ESM should reveal less resistance of the tissues indicating that there has been a favorable response to the treatment.

This is a description of the soft tissue technique called the "ileus prevention treatment." This technique has been proven[2] in the clinical arena, preventing and treating postoperative ileus.

C. ABDOMINAL COLLATERAL GANGLIA:

There are three main sympathetic collateral ganglia in the abdominal area; these are the celiac, the superior mesenteric, and the inferior mesenteric ganglia. These ganglia are located in the immediate preaortic area and posterior to an imaginary line drawn from the xiphoid process to the umbilicus.

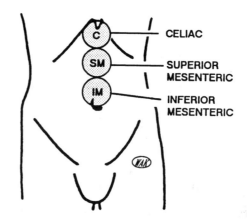

The celiac ganglion is usually separated into a right and a left ganglion. Functionally the celiac ganglion innervates the upper GI tract (stomach, duodenum, liver, gallbladder, pancreas and spleen). The superior mesenteric ganglion is located around the base of the superior mesenteric artery and innervates the entire small intestine below the duodenum, the right side of the colon, and also the kidneys, adrenals and the gonads. The inferior mesenteric ganglion, located around the base of the inferior mesenteric artery, supplies the left colon and the pelvic organs (except for the gonads).

DIAGNOSIS OF FACILITATION OF AN ABDOMINAL COLLATERAL GANGLION:

o .. The extended fingers of both hands are placed over the midline of the abdomen between the xiphoid process and the umbilicus

o .. The longer fingers are bent slightly to produce fingers of equal length and therefore fingers that will make equal depth of penetration when pressure is applied

o .. Objective sensation of a rapid increase in residence as pressure is directed by extended fingers applied against the abdominal wall and directly over the ganglion

o .. Subjective complaint of increased tenderness with mild to moderate pressure

o .. Positive responses to questioning of the patient regarding signs and symptoms related to the organ or organs innervated by the tender ganglion

GANGLION INHIBITION TREATMENT TECHNIQUE:

o .. The extended fingers of both hands are placed over the midline of the abdomen and over the tender involved (facilitated) ganglion

o .. The longer fingers are bent slightly to produce fingers of equal length and therefore fingers that will make equal depth of penetration when pressure is applied

o .. The patient takes a half-breath in against the operator's finger resistance and holds it as long as possible

o .. With exhalation, the operator follows the tissues in until a new point of resistence is met; the breathing cycle is repeated

o .. Posterior pressure is applied and increased to a point where the resistance is evident and the pressure is tolerable to the patient

o .. This pressure is held until the relaxation of resistance is experienced by the physician or the pressure has been maintained for about 90 seconds.

o .. Recheck diagnostic pressure over the ganglion should indicate significant reduction in subjective complaint and a palpable reduction in tissue resistance

D. CHAPMAN'S REFLEXES: DIAGNOSIS

Chapman's reflexes were recorded by Owen in a book entitled Chapman Reflexes: Owen's Endocrine Interpretation. The points seem better related to the sympathetic system than to the endocrine system. Chapman charted anterior and posterior myofascial points where tenderness to mild to moderate pressure was related to organ dysfunction in a predictable organ. (See charts on pages 232 and 233). Like any diagnostic system, positive findings in this non-invasive system of diagnosis must be correlated and interpreted with other

200

historical and physical findings of visceral dysfunction. Their presence should also be correlated with other findings of sympathetic hyperactivity. Since the anterior points are more sensitive and more spread out than posterior points, they are usually used for diagnosis and the posterior points are used for treatment. A tender anterior Chapman point indicates a possible organ dysfunction requiring further history and physical evaluation. The anterior points are also used to evaluate the success of treatment of that organ dysfunction or disease.

Diagnostically, Chapman's reflex points should be sought prior to any manipulative treatment which might modify their presence. Most physicians use the anterior Chapman points for an aid to diagnosis of systemic diseases but do not use the original Chapman treatment techniques.

CHAPMAN'S REFLEXES: TREATMENT

In the original Chapman method,[3] after treating pelvic somatic dysfunction, the posterior points were treated first using a circular type of soft tissue manipulation. The anterior points were only used for treatment if the posterior treatment was unsuccessful. Some physicians proposed that the treatment of all points related to the same visceral system be utilized to enhance homeostatic function of that system.

Using the original treatment method, posterior Chapman's points were treated by performing circular soft tissue treatment over the tender posterior point for 20 to 30 seconds. The anterior Chapman's points are usually too tender to treat with this soft tissue procedure. The anterior tibial bands (relating to the colon) are an exception to this. These points are very susceptible to circular soft tissue or rapid mechanical pressure to produce reflex autonomic normalization in the colon for such syndromes as irritable bowel syndrome, post-viral diarrhea and ulcerative colitis.

Posterior myofascial points by Chapman were treated with a circular soft tissue technique to produce reflex changes in the viscera and improve organ function. This is effective, but the paraspinal soft tissue used by most osteopathic physicians during their manipulative management of a patient produces similar results and could be directed to the areas of somatic change. Charts of Chapman's reflexes are available through the Department of Osteopathic Theory and Methods at the Kirksville College of Osteopathic Medicine.[4]

E. THE CERVICAL GANGLIA:

The cervical sympathetic ganglia are not in the thoracolumbar outflow and they certainly do not fit into the rib raising mechanisms; but they are important in sympathetic responses in the body, especially the heart and structures of the head (sinuses) and neck. Eight original cervical paraspinal ganglia have coalesced to form 2 or 3 cervical ganglia (the superior, middle, and sometimes the inferior). They would be just like any other paraspinal ganglia except that the cell bodies for these cervical ganglia are located at spinal levels T1-4.

The inferior cervical ganglion lies on the ventral surface of the head of the first rib and is frequently fused with the first thoracic ganglion to form the stellate ganglion. It serves C7, C8, and T1 (and sometimes C6). The middle cervical ganglion lies approximately at the level of the C6 vertebra and has connections with C5 and C6 (and sometimes C4 and C7). The superior cervical ganglion is a long ganglion that lies anterior to the transverse processes of C2, C3, and C4 and sends sympathetic fibers to cervical nerves C1-4. Each of the three cervical ganglia sends a cardiac nerve to one of the cardiac plexuses.

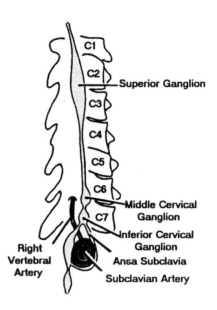

The fascias around these ganglia are closely related to the cervical joints and the fascial planes of the neck. The cervical ganglia and their activity can be compromised by somatic dysfunction in the cervical joints or by abnormal tensions in the cervical fascias. Sinusitis, ear or eye dysfunctions, cardiac tachyarrhythmias, and other cardiac dysfunctions may be altered by freeing cervical pathways and treating cervical joint somatic dysfunctions. This is especially true in the C1-4 and the cervicothoracic junction areas.

III. TREATMENT FOR LYMPHATIC SYSTEM DYSFUNCTION:

A. BASICS: Goals of Treatment and General Manipulative Treatment Plan:

o .. To promote the free flow of lymph through its lymphatic vessels and fascial pathways. These pathways extend from interstitial tissue spaces to the venous circulation in the upper chest via the right and left lymphatic ducts.

o .. To improve function of the abdominal diaphragm, the extrinsic pump for the lymphatic system.

o .. To reduce sympathetic outflow.

o .. The cervicothoracic diaphragm is a common pathway in the course of lymph drainage from any place in the body. For this reason, the thoracic inlet is diagnosed for fascial rotational preference and treated as indicated.

o .. Tensions in fascial planes and the other regional myofascial diaphragms located at the junctions of structural change also hinder the flow of lymph. For this reason, the other three fascial and muscular diaphragms may be diagnosed and treated as indicated (craniocervical, abdominal and pelvic).

The paraspinal musculature at the thoracolumbar junction is relaxed by soft tissue, stretching, and/or myofascial treatments. The abdominal diaphragm is then redomed.

The pelvic diaphragm works synchronously and passively with the abdominal diaphragm to produce optimal pressure gradients between the thoracic and abdominal cavities.

o .. Lymphatic pump techniques are used to encourage lymphatic flow through the pathways

o .. Rib raising in areas of major venous and lymphatic vessels is often necessary because hypersympathetic tone will constrict the larger veins promoting congestion of tissues in that vein's region of drainage; hypersympathetic tone also constricts the larger lymphatic vessels and restricts the drainage of lymph from their regions.

B. SYMPTOMS OF FASCIAL DYSFUNCTION:

POSTURAL SYMPTOMS:

Whenever there is dysfunction or disease, the body's tissues and systems must participate in the establishment of a new homeostatic level for body function. The type, severity and site of the stress determines which systems will need to compensate the most; the neuromusculoskeletal system is involved in all dysfunctions and disease processes.

Postural diagnosis provides an uncomplicated, non-invasive access to the obvious expression of the function of the entire person. Structurally, the AP and lateral curves are affected by gravity. Lateral curves may develop and are particularly affected by inequality of the sacral base from such conditions as a short leg or a sacral shear, or from an unlevel cranial base as may occur with birth injury or certain somatic dysfunctions in this region. When no cause for scoliosis is found its etiology is termed idiopathic; Osteopathic recognition of these postural causes allows re-classification of some previously diagnosed idiopathic scolioses. Rotational curvatures are often maintained by regional fascial plane rotations or torsions. It is well known that the emotions may be mirrored in the posture of a person. It has been clinically observed that postural imbalance which initially affects any one of the three cardinal planes of the body will also affect the remaining two body planes and the total posture of the patient.

A "short leg" may result from a congenital developmental defect or it can be produced by a leg fracture, by muscle spasm, or by physiologic or nonphysiologic joint somatic dysfunctions. Sometimes the myofascial compensation is so good that a spine appears to be straight even when there is a very obvious short leg. With time, however, the person will develop lateral scoliotic curvatures of the spine. Since sidebending motion of the spine is always accompanied by rotation, these lateral curves are often said to exhibit rotoscoliosis.

SYSTEMIC CHANGES:

In the supine position, normally the motion generated by quiet breathing should be observed "down to the pubic symphysis." Failure to observe this in a patient suggests that the diaphragm is not contracting from a well-domed starting position, is contracting poorly, or is demonstrating asymmetrical of contraction between the right and left hemidiaphragm. Poor respiratory function results in a wide range of congestive symptoms which vary some depending upon which tissues or system of tissues are congested. Healthy tissue and good function depends upon adequate circulation and removal of excessive interstitial fluids from the tissues and their return to the venous system and the heart. Venous and lymphatic drainage depend on good abdominal diaphragmatic action and effective pressure gradients between the abdominal and thoracic cavities. Examples of symptoms and signs from various areas of congestion are listed below:

PELVIS	LEGS	HEAD (CNS)
hemorrhoids varicosities	edema night cramps	malaise confusion dizziness
SPINE (CNS)	**BOWEL**	nausea irritability
Backaches	constipation	headaches

204

Whenever fascias are subjected to prolonged abnormal physical or chemical stress they become thickened and reinforced by fibroblastic activity. The large non-aqueous molecules of the interstitial edema will also stimulate fibroproliferation and subsequent fibrosis if it they are not properly reabsorbed. Fibrosis shortens the supporting tissues and impairs joint and general body motions. The chronic pull of shortened fascias on bony attachments may result in excessive proliferation of bone called spurs which can be seen on x-ray. Chronic congestion also results in contractures and/or calcification as well as generally compromising the intercellular environment of the tissues involved.

OTHER SYMPTOMS AND SIGNS OF FASCIAL DYSFUNCTION:

fascial preference	tissue congestion	thickened fascias
tissue contracture	restricted motion	ticklishness
tenderness	shortness of breath	faulty posture
poor circulation	myofascial points	strains/sprains
limitation of motion	trophic skin changes	muscle cramps

```
"not breathing down to the pubes"
costal breathing by a relaxed person
increased lumbar lordosis in the supine relaxed patient
pain on palpation over fascial dysfunction especially near
   areas of fascial attachments, at points of fascial
   calcification, and where forces of stress converge
general fatigue or malaise with no physical or laboratory
   tests indicate disease.
```

C. DIAGNOSTIC AREAS INDICATING REGIONAL TISSUE CONGESTION:

Because of the arrangement of regional lymphatic and venous drainage channels, fascial stress is revealed in body fascial patterns, preferences in regional fascial plane motion and congestive changes in the soft tissues, especially in spinal areas where there is a change in structure or function from one region to the next.

Tissue congestion in certain key areas of the body provide a clue to congestive dysfunction in designated body regions. Regional congestion can be suspected by palpating tissue texture changes at these specific sites.

o .. Bogginess or edema in the supraclavicular area indicates evidence of tissue congestion from poor lymphatic drainage and dysfunction somewhere in the head and neck.

205

o .. Fullness and tenderness on palpation of the posterior axillary fold indicates congestion, poor lymphatic drainage, and dysfunction somewhere in the upper extremity.

o .. Bogginess in the epigastric area around the xiphoid process means congestion, poor lymphatic drainage, and dysfunction somewhere in the abdomen.

o .. Bogginess in the inguinal area means congestion, poor lymphatic drainage, and dysfunction somewhere in the lower extremity.

o .. Bogginess in the popliteal space--problem is in the knee, leg, or foot.

o .. Bogginess just anterior to Achilles tendon or thickening of the Achilles tendon itself--problem is in the ankle or foot.

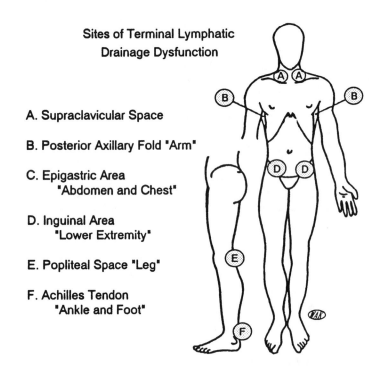

Sites of Terminal Lymphatic
Drainage Dysfunction

A. Supraclavicular Space

B. Posterior Axillary Fold "Arm"

C. Epigastric Area
"Abdomen and Chest"

D. Inguinal Area
"Lower Extremity"

E. Popliteal Space "Leg"

F. Achilles Tendon
"Ankle and Foot"

Inhalation, with contraction of the abdominal diaphragm, produces negative intrathoracic pressure and positive intra-abdominal pressure because of fascial compartmentalization. With diaphragmatic relaxation, intrathoracic pressure is relatively increased and intra-abdominal pressure is relatively decreased. This reciprocal action of the diaphragm produces pressure gradients between the two cavities of the body and along with the one-way valves in the veins and large lymphatic vessels, aids venous return and provides an extrinsic pump mechanism for the movement of lymph through the lymphatic vessels, back to the central circulation and the heart.

Diaphragmatic action is most efficient when the diaphragm is well domed, its nerve supply via the phrenic nerve (C3, 4, 5) is not compromised, and the lymphatic pathways are unhindered. Fascial restrictions and torsions of fascial pathways and diaphragms can lead to passive congestion and dysfunction of the lymphatics, the lungs, and other body systems and tissues.

> **Clinical Principle:** The most common site for relative obstruction to lymphatic flow, no matter what tissue of the body is congested, is the fascial diaphragm at the thoracic inlet, the cervicothoracic diaphragm (Sibson's fascia).

D. FASCIAL PATTERNS FOR DIAGNOSIS OF REGIONAL FASCIAL DYSFUNCTION:

Fascias are affected by a person's structural and functional stresses even when that person believes that he/she is healthy. Gravity is one of the significant natural stressors affecting upright body posture; and the fascias can be examined for evidence of compromised homeostatic mechanisms.

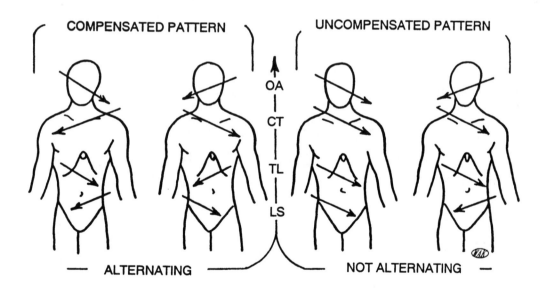

FASCIAL PATTERNS
ACCORDING TO GORDON ZINK, D.O.

J. Gordon Zink, D.O., FAAO, (formerly at the University of Osteopathic Medicine and Health Sciences at Des Moines, Iowa) popularized the use of fascial diagnosis and treatment. Zink had clinically studied postural patterns and observed that almost all of the people who thought that they were well had alternating fascial patterns rather than the ideal, in which no fascial preference was palpated. Fascial direction alternated at anatomical "transition" sites: the occipitoatlantal area, the cervicothoracic area, the thoracolumbar area, and the lumbosacral area. Alternation of fascial patterns is a homeostatic postural response providing compensation when the ideal cannot be reached.

Alternating patterns are termed compensatory fascial patterns. Zink then found that 80% of the "well people" had a particular compensatory pattern in which there was preference for its rotation to the left at the occipitoatlantal area, to the right at the cervicothoracic area, to the left at the thoracolumbar area and to the right at the lumbosacral area (i.e. left/right/left/right or L,R,L,R). Because this pattern was so common he named it the "Common Compensatory Pattern (CCP)" and the clinicians often add the words, "of Zink" in recognition of his contribution.

Most of the 20% remaining who thought they were well also had a compensated fascial pattern but it was just the opposite of the Common Compensatory Pattern. The motion preference of the fascias at the four reference areas in these subjects was right/left/right/left (i.e. R/L/R/L). Dr. Zink termed this the "uncommon compensatory pattern."

Those people who do not have the ideal fascial pattern and who are not homeostatically capable of reaching one of the compensatory patterns are said to have an uncompensated fascial pattern. This means that fascial preferences do not alternate in direction from one reference area to the next. Non-compensated patterns often have a traumatic origin.

Rather than list the preferred fascial plane motion at each area when recording structural findings on a physical examination or talking to someone about a person's fascial patterns, the student or physician may write or state something like one of the following:

o .. the fascial pattern is ideal.

o .. the fascial pattern is in the common compensatory pattern of Zink.

o .. according to the Zink patterns, the fascia is out of the CCP at...(and then names the area or areas that do not fit the CCP.)

o .. the uncommon compensatory pattern according to Zink is present..

Dr. Zink observed that if a person's fascias fit the ideal pattern (equal preference to sidebending and rotation right and left in all of these body areas or had one of the compensatory patterns identified as the CCP of L,R,L,R rotations respectively or the uncommon compensatory pattern of R,L,R,L), they tolerated stress, somatic dysfunction, illness, and disease better, responded to medical care more predictably, and recovered quicker and more completely than persons who had an uncompensated fascial pattern.

E. THE FASCIAL DIAPHRAGMS, OTHER PATHWAYS, AND THEIR TREATMENTS:

SOFT TISSUE DIAGNOSIS OF THE THORACIC INLET:

The anatomical thoracic inlet is defined as being outlined by the manubrium, the right and left first rib and the first thoracic vertebra. The functional thoracic inlet is the clinical thoracic inlet and is defined as being the manubrium with the angle of Louis, the first two ribs on each side and the first four thoracic vertebrae. When an osteopathic physician talks about the thoracic inlet he/she almost always means this functional thoracic inlet.

This diagram illustrates the thoracic inlet and illustrates the important static landmarks that are used in the diagnosis of fascial rotational preference (torsion) of the thoracic inlet.

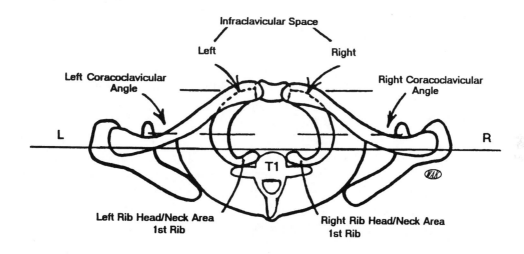

The thoracic inlet is divided into two parts by the mediastinum with the remaining spaces (one on each side of the mediastinum) providing an opening through which the apex of the right and left lungs project upward into the cervical area to a height of about 2.5-3 cm above the clavicles. The apices of the lungs and the thoracic inlet are covered by Sibson's fascia.

These thick cupolae are formed from fascias from the longus coli muscle deep in the cervicothoracic area and from the fascias on the inner surfaces of the scalenus anticus, medius and posticus muscles laterally. Both the left and the right lymphatic ducts of the body must pass through this diaphragm. The rotational preference of these fascias should be evaluated mechanically whenever there is an upset of fluid homeostasis anywhere in the body.

The thoracic duct (the left lymphatic duct) passes through the cervicothoracic diaphragm once, travels 3-4 cm up into the neck to a level approximately lateral to the left transverse process of the C7 vertebra, makes a U-turn, and comes back down through this fascial diaphragm the second time into the thoracic cage where it empties into the venous system at the junction of the left subclavian and left internal jugular veins. The right lymphatic duct also passes through the thoracic inlet, but only once. (The site at which the lymphatic ducts empty into the venous system may vary slightly. They enter into the region of the brachiocephalic vein.)

When palpating the thoracic inlet of a seated patient, the palpating fingers must be close enough to the vertebral column at T1 so that they are over the costovertebral and costotransverse area of the first rib. Is one side higher than the other? If one rib head seems to be elevated in relation to the other, it may indicate somatic dysfunction of the first rib. It may also mean that the fascias of the cervicothoracic junction (the thoracic inlet) are holding the cervicothoracic region of the body, sidebent and rotated to the side opposite the elevated rib. The first thoracic vertebra may also exhibit a neutral type somatic dysfunction which will be sidebent to the opposite side and rotated to the same side. In all of these cases, the rib head will be tender to the patient on the side of the palpable "elevated rib head;" differential diagnosis is then necessary.

If the infraclavicular spaces near the manubrium are equal in depth, there could be an elevated rib or the first thoracic vertebra could be sidebent to the opposite side, producing a secondary elevation of the first rib head. If the infraclavicular space is more shallow on the same side as the elevated first rib head then a rotational fascial preference of the thoracic inlet is present.

Examples: (x = one direction and y is the opposite direction)

An elevated and tender first rib on side x and a shallow infraclavicular space on side x indicates that the fascial pattern of the thoracic inlet is sidebent and rotated y.

An elevated and tender first rib on side x with an equal depth to the infraclavicular spaces on side x and y, indicates that this is not due to fascial dysfunction of the thoracic inlet. These changes could mean an elevated first rib on side x or/and a neutral type first thoracic vertebral somatic dysfunction with sidebending y.

As with all diagnoses of somatic dysfunction, motion testing is the final and most reliable verification.

The thoracic inlet of a patient whose general body fascias are in the Common Compensatory Pattern of Zink will have the left first rib elevated and the right infraclavicular space will be deeper (the left infraclavicular space near the sternum more shallow).

The apex of the coracoclavicular angle on the left will be more anterior than on the right. The following diagram illustrates the fascial rotational preference of the thoracic inlet as it would be found in a patient whose total body fascial pattern agrees with the CCP of Zink.

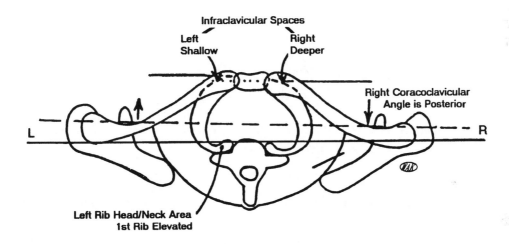

It is important to remember that the fascial patterns from all of the four junctional areas must be diagnosed before one knows if any one fascial pattern is in agreement with a compensated or uncompensated pattern. The following diagram illustrates fascial patterns that are pulling the inlet into sidebending left and rotation left as would be found in a patient who had the other patterns compatible with the uncommon compensatory pattern of Zink.

211

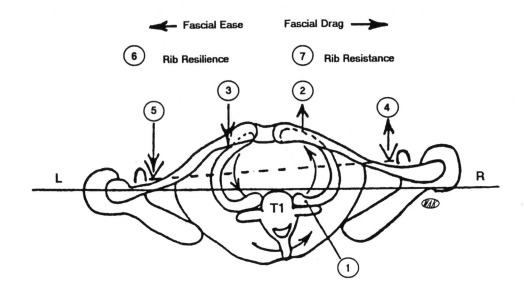

Fascial Ease ←   Fascial Drag →

6   Rib Resilience   7   Rib Resistance

MANIPULATIVE TREATMENT OF THE THORACIC INLET (CERVICOTHORACIC DIAPHRAGM):

MANIPULATION OF THE THORACIC INLET WITH INDIRECT MYOFASCIAL UNWINDING TREATMENT:

o .. The patient may be sitting or supine.
o .. The operator's hands bridge each shoulder with the fingers anterior and the thumbs posterior.
o .. The tissues are followed in their preference for sidebending and rotation and held in that position as the patient breaths in and out.
o .. The operator follows the tissue preferences until the tissues approach the midline again.

MANIPULATION OF THE THORACIC INLET BY TWO-STEP DIRECT TECHNIQUE:

o .. The patient is supine.

Step One (correction of sidebending component):

o .. The operator's MP joint of one hand is placed at the posterolateral cervicothoracic junction and will be used as a fulcrum for direct method sidebending.
o .. The head and neck is taken as a unit and sidebent to the restrictive barrier.
o .. The patient's head is turned to the opposite side to lock the cervical spine.
o .. Adjustment of the sagittal plane localizes the forces at the cervicothoracic junction and a thrust is carried through the fulcrum hand toward the opposite axilla while the cephalic hand counters the sidebending thrust. (Rx sidebending component)

Step Two (correction of rotational component):

o .. A fulcrum is placed at the cervicothoracic junction (CT) on the other side and the head and neck is rotated to the rotational barrier at the cervicothoracic inlet, without sidebending the neck.
o .. The sagittal plane and sometimes a slight sidebending adjustment is made to localize well and a rotational thrust is made through the rotational barrier at the CT junction.

MANIPULATION OF THE THORACIC INLET IN SITTING ONE STEP TECHNIQUE:

o .. The patient is sitting.
o .. The operator's hand on the side of the patient's somatic dysfunction is placed on the patient's shoulder.
o .. The operator's foot on the side opposite the somatic dysfunction is placed on the table next to the patient and the patient's arm on that side is draped over the operator's thigh.
o .. The operator's thumb is placed on the spinous process of T1, the opposite hand is placed along side the patient's head and neck on the opposite side, and the patient's head is sidebent toward the side of the CT somatic dysfunction; the head is extended to localize and the patient's body is directed into a posterior and sidebent away position by guidance through the operator's knee.
o .. When all forces are localized there is a thrust with the thumb on the T1 spinous process away from the side of somatic dysfunction (this reverses the rotation) and at the same time, (because of position of the patient's neck) sidebending is reversed.

DIAGNOSIS AND TREATMENT OF THE ABDOMINAL DIAPHRAGM

DIAGNOSIS OF THE THORACOABDOMINAL DIAPHRAGM (THE EXTRINSIC PUMP FOR THE LYMPHATIC SYSTEM):

The thoracoabdominal diaphragm at the thoracolumbar region (TL) is the main extrinsic pump for the lymphatic system. Diaphragmatic dysfunction is suspected when respiratory effort does not produce movement of the abdominal tissues down to the level of the pubic symphysis. Elements of this dysfunction can be diagnosed indirectly through the fascias using one flat hand in the epigastric area and the posterior hand at the thoracolumbar junction to examine for palpatory preference of rotation about an anterior/posterior (AP) axis. Other elements can be diagnosed by directly attempting to rotate the thoracolumbar "tube" right and then left. Once the diagnosis of the myofascial preference is known, treatment can be effectively applied. Lasting effect from a redoming manipulative technique to the thoracoabdominal diaphragm often depends on removing dysfunction of its attachments and functional extensions. This includes proper treatment of somatic dysfunction of L1-3, the lower six ribs, and reduction of lumbar lordosis. The role of quadratus lumborum dysfunction in inhibiting the effectiveness of these techniques should be noted and it is important to remember that the diaphragm is innervated by the phrenic nerve, C3,4,5. It seems prudent to manipulate any somatic dysfunction found in the lumbars, lower ribs, quadratus lumborum muscle, pelvis, and the iliopsoas muscle first.

MANIPULATIVE TREATMENT IN PREPARATION FOR DIAPHRAGM REDOMING:

If there is increased tone in the thoracolumbar paraspinal musculature and increased lumbar lordosis, utilize any and all methods of soft tissue kneading, stretch, and/or myofascial treatment to relax the region.

TREATMENT FOR QUADRATUS LUMBORUM SPASM OR LUMBAR PARAVERTEBRAL MUSCLE SPASM:

The primary intent of treatment is to stretch the quadratus lumborum and re-establish normal 12th rib motion. The following example of a direct method treatment uses respiratory cooperation of the patient.

o .. The patient is prone; the arm on the side of dysfunction is resting by the side of the head.
o .. The lower extremities are moved to the edge of the table away from the side of myofascial dysfunction.

o .. The operator stands on the side opposite the dysfunction and contacts the shaft of the 12th rib with the full length of the thumb on the cephalic hand, to stabilize the rib.

o .. The pelvis is grasped with the fingers of the caudal hand by curling the fingers around the anterior superior iliac spine (ASIS).

o .. The operator's contacts are separated by lifting the pelvis and carrying the rib anterior and superior.

o .. The patient is instructed to inhale as the operator maintains tension at the contacts. Muscle energy is applied by having the patient pull the ASIS toward the table against resistance.

o .. Traction/separation is increased to take up slack when the patient exhales and relaxes; the same procedure with respiratory cooperation is repeated.

Stretching of the quadratus lumborum can also be performed with the patient in the lateral recumbent position. With the patient in this position, the side of dysfunction is up and there is a pillow under the opposite side. Increased stretch can be achieved by dropping the patient's feet off the side of the table.

Sometimes, spray and stretch of quadratus lumborum myofascial trigger point(s), as described by Travell, is necessary in recurrent or recalcitrant dysfunction.[5]

ILIOPSOAS RELEASE TREATMENT:

See Jones Strain/Counterstrain indirect method for treatment applicable to acute situations. Example: The lower extremities of the supine patient are flexed externally rotated, and sidebent until 70% or more of the subjective tenderness over the iliacus counterstrain point is relieved. This position is held 90 seconds and then passively returned to a neutral position. If not acute, direct stretch using muscle energy and exercise is very appropriate.

DIRECT (STRETCH) METHOD TREATMENT OF THE ABDOMINAL DIAPHRAGM:

o .. The patient is supine and the operator stands at the head or at the side of the table

o .. The margins of the lower rib cage are gently grasped and pulled and/or pushed to its rotation restriction and held as the patient deeply breathes in and out

o .. Sometimes a superior or inferior vector is added to the direct rotation of the thoracic cage so that there is good palpable movement of both sides of the diaphragm during deep breathing, i.e. both leaves of the diaphragm are moving well.

o .. This position is held for about three big breaths so that the fascial preference is eliminated and the respiratory effort has redomed the diaphragm.

INDIRECT METHOD OF TREATMENT FOR THE ABDOMINAL DIAPHRAGM:

o .. The patient is supine and the operator stands at the side of the table.
o .. The operator's caudal hand is placed on the abdomen with the fingers immediately below the xiphoid process (the anterior attachment of the abdominal diaphragm); the cephalad hand contacts and bridges the paraspinal regions from L1-3 (posterior attachment of the abdominal diaphragm).
o .. The operator's caudal hand produces clockwise and counterclockwise motion in the abdominal fascias to determine direction of fascial freedom.
o .. The abdominal fascias are held in the direction of freedom with one hand and the fascias of the paraspinal tissues at the thoracolumbar junction are held in the opposite direction. The tissues are balanced in this position until release is appreciated.

DIAGNOSIS AND MANIPULATIVE TECHNIQUES OF THE PELVIC DIAPHRAGM:

The pelvic diaphragm is diagnosed by pressing extended fingers into the lateral side of the ischiorectal fossa; or placing the thumbs into the upper posterolateral margin of the ischiorectal fossa; or through evaluation of the muscles of the pelvic diaphragm during a rectal or vaginal examination. The pelvic diaphragm can be treated through the perineum, through the rectum, or through the vagina. Daily pelvic coil or Kegel exercises by the patient at home helps to maintain pelvic tone after a successful manipulative treatment.

ISCHIORECTAL FOSSA TREATMENT: (a fascial release treatment)

o .. The patient is lateral recumbent with the fossa to be treated away from the table; or the patient could be supine. In either of these positions, the patient has the hips and knees flexed 90 degrees. The patient could be prone but in that position the hips could not be flexed 90 degrees.
o .. The operator stands behind the table or at the foot of the table, identifies the ischial tuberosity and the coccyx, and then uses the extended fingers to contact the lateral margin of that ischiorectal fossa (the interphalangeal joints are fully extended and the metacarpophalangeal joints slightly flexed; the wrist is held rigid).
o .. The operator sometimes sits on the table and braces the elbow aginst his/her own ilium.

o .. The operator's cephalic hand may be placed on the patient's hip for counterforce.

o .. The fingertips are gently inserted to compress the fat of the fossa as far as allowed by the fascias and as is tolerated by the patient.

o .. Tension (and direction of treatment) will be slightly more *posterior* if rectal problems are present, more *anterior* (but still in the ischiorectal fossa) if bladder problems are present, and just *superior* if ovarian and/or broad ligament congestion is present.

o .. The patient is asked to breathe in and exhale; the fingers drift more superiorly as the fingers follow the diaphragm with exhalation; the push of the pelvic diaphragm is resisted when the patient inhales.

INTRAVAGINAL FASCIAL RELEASE:

o .. The muscle and fascia of the pelvic diaphragm and their areas of tension are identified by sweeping laterally over the pelvic wall.

o .. The fingers are spread in the transverse plane of the vagina to hold the orifice open

o .. The patient is then asked to cough sharply 2 or 3 times and the fascia and pelvic muscular diaphragm are automatically stretched by contact with the operator's fingers.

o .. The pelvic diaphragm is again palpated to evaluate the treatment's effect on the tense tissues.

INTRARECTAL FASCIAL RELEASE: The principles for stretch of pelvic diaphragm are similar to those used in the intravaginal treatment but are carried out through the rectum using a single gloved finger and a good lubricant. The pelvic diaphragm is palpable through the rectal wall and the location of tension is mentally recorded. Cough is not used to activate; rather, the fingers press firmly and steadily without hurting the patient, until relaxation of the pelvic diaphragm is palpable.

MANIPULATION OF THE CRANIAL DIAPHRAGM:

Not all physicians are able to utilize cranial diagnosis and treatment; but condylar decompression and muscle energy to stretch the OA fascia can be performed easily by any physician with manipulative skills.

Diagnosis and cranial treatment can be studied by taking specific undergraduate or postgraduate courses in this field. An important reference text is Harold Magoun's book, Osteopathy in the Cranial Field. Contact the Sutherland Cranial Teaching Foundation, the American Academy of Osteopathy or the Cranial Academy for postgraduate CME courses.

IV. OTHER SOFT TISSUE TREATMENTS TO AID IN LYMPHATIC DRAINAGE

LYMPHATIC PUMP TECHNIQUES:

THE GOALS OF LYMPHATIC PUMP PROCEDURES:

o .. to accentuate negative intrathoracic pressure
o .. to increase venous and lymphatic return
o .. to increase homeostasis (immune function)
o .. to mobilize fluids
o .. to mobilize thick plugs of mucus (vibratory treatment)

TREATMENT WITH USE OF LYMPHATIC PUMPS:

THORACIC LYMPHATIC PUMP TREATMENT: This works by increasing the positive pressure in the chest through direct pressure on the chest alternating with negative pressure which is increased by the release of this chest pressure.

o .. The patient is passively supine throughout the entire treatment with the head turned slightly aside to avoid breathing in the operator's face.
o .. The operator stands at the head of the patient and applies both hands to the sides of the patient's chest cage bilaterally (usually in the upper ribs at about the mid-clavicular line).
o .. A steady pressure is applied during the patient's exhalation phase; this is directed in a functional pattern for the ribs to aid in exhalation. A vibratory component may be added during exhalation to assist in moving secretions.
o .. The application and release may be rhythmic at about 90-120 times per minute; or the operator may hold pressure until shortly after the patient initiates a breath and then suddenly release the chest pressure (this last method is repeated with each exhalation/inhalation of the patient). The operator must be sure that the patient does not have gum, candy or loose dentures in the mouth.

> **IMPORTANT:** If the patient is very short of breath (as in COPD), their own intrinsic rate of respiration should not be disturbed. In more vital patients, this procedure is optimally performed with a rhythm or while directing the patient through the exhalation and inhalation portions of the cycle.

PEDAL LYMPHATIC PUMP (DALYRIMPLE): This technique works through fascial pumps and by the massage of the diaphragm (and indirectly the lung bases) utilizing the intermittent movement of the abdominal contents up against the diaphragm. This "intermittent motion" aids in increasing the range of positive/negative pressure gradients.

o .. The patient is passively supine throughout the treatment
o .. The operator stands at the patient's feet and intermittently and rhythmically applies activating force through the feet at a rate determined by watching the reaction of the patient's abdomen. A rate of 90-120/min is common.

> Dorsiflexion of the feet with the operator's hand on the plantar surfaces and the fingers over the toes stretches the posterior fascias of the leg and is primarily directed into the lumbar and lumbosacral regions.

> Plantar flexion of the feet stretches the anterior fascias and is directed primarily to the thoracic region, ribs, and cervical areas.

PECTORAL TRACTION: This works by helping to elevate the first 6-7 ribs during inhalation and thereby increasing the negative pressure during that phase of respiration. Two minutes of pectoralis traction treatment is believed to provide as much assistance to lymphatic flow as five minutes of thoracic pump treatment.

o .. The patient is supine with knees drawn up and hands on the abdomen.
o .. The operator is at the head of the patient and gently grasps the anterior axillary fold (pectoralis muscles) with the fingers carefully conforming to the patient and not gouging.
o .. Gentle traction is applied in a medial, anterior and cephalic direction and held for 1-3 minutes while the patient breathes normally or with slight increase in volume. The grasp is reapplied as needed to permit patient comfort.

> Family members can be taught this method of moving fluids with relative safety compared to some of the other techniques described in this section.

SPLENIC PUMP:

This technique is effective in patients with systemic infections and anemic patients with low resistance to infection. The spleen stores red and white cells and screens the blood of damaged blood cells.

o .. The patient is supine; the operator stands on the left side and places his/her hands opposite each other on the lower left rib cage.
o .. Gentle alternate compression and release is applied until tissues release. The amount of pressure depends upon the patient's condition and the judgement of the physician. Avoid in cases with friable splenomegaly.

LIVER PUMP:

This procedure is performed much the same as the splenic pump except it is applied over the liver. The liver has a rich bed of lymphatic vessels. Its decongestion aids in detoxification and helps to relieve visceral congestion.

POSTERIOR AXILLARY FOLD TECHNIQUE:

The goal is to reduce local tenderness and induration in the myofascial tissues of the posterior axillary fold; if the patient is able to sense the warmth that accompanies good lymph flow, the desire is to treat so that the "warmth" encompasses the entire arm to the fingers. Concomitant myofascial trigger points in the posterior axillary fold may also be addressed with this technique.

o .. patient supine and operator facing the patient
o .. grasp superior portion of the posterior axillary fold with thumb anteriorly and the index, middle and ring fingers posteriorly, both the thumb and fingers are next to chest wall
o .. apply steady, gentle but firm squeeze pressure for 10-15 seconds and inquire about "sensation of warmth in fingers or arm"
o .. if warmth is sensed by the patient, it can be accentuated by having the patient clench and unclench the fist to accentuate the peripheral muscular lymphatic pumps.

LOWER EXTREMITY FASCIAL PATHWAY TREATMENT:

o .. patient is supine with the treatment leg off the table and knee bent
o .. the operator straddles the leg just above the ankle and grasps the patient's leg by clasping the hands together just below the knee joint (thumbs are often right over the medial and lateral margins of the joint space)
o .. operator leans backward applying gentle upward, outward, caudal and rotational encouragement until the forces are centered (stacked in all motions) at the femoroacetabular joint, knee and ankle. This technique frees the fascial pathways of the leg, thigh, and hip and improves lymphatic flow from the lower extremity.
o .. if the patient is able to sense the warmth that accompanies good lymph flow, it should gradually move to the foot; if the warmth does not progress, specific OMT to that site would be beneficial.

VENTRAL ABDOMINAL MANIPULATIVE TECHNIQUES:

ASCENDING AND DESCENDING COLON MESENTERIC RELEASE:
The accessible parts of the colon are palpated to detect tension increases, congestion, and/or restriction in the motion of their mesenteries. In these techniques, the bowel is gently taken at right angles toward its mesenteric attachments and to the extent allowed by its motion barrier. Gentle tension is then applied to its attachments. The technique is activated by having the patient take a shallow breath and hold it until a breath is needed. When the patient has to breathe again there will be a slight give to the mesentery. This technique is repeated 2-3 times.

RELEASE OF AN ENTRAPPED CECUM:

o .. the patient is supine and the operator at the patient's side
o .. the patient's knee is slightly bent on the right side to relax the abdominal musculature over the cecum
o .. the operator applies the heel of his/her right hand to the right lower quadrant of the abdomen (RLQ) of the abdomen
o .. the operator attempts to gently lift the cecum from the pelvic entrapment and toward the hepatic flexure of the colon
o .. the opposite hand (optimal) may be used for inhibition to the thoracolumbar junction where cecal sympathetic cell bodies of the spinal cord are located

This technique is a slow maneuver allowing for release of the cecum from its entrapment in the pelvis. The patient may complain of fullness and some pain in the ascending colon as well as the hepatic flexure as the operator's right hand releases the entrapment and moves the fecal mass and intestinal gas along the ascending colon.

ABDOMINAL MESENTERIC FASCIAL RELEASES:

o .. the patient is supine; the operator stands on the side of his dominant eye and facing partially toward the head of the table
o .. starting at the right lower quadrant (RLQ), the operator uses one hand on top of the other to gently move the abdominal wall and the underlying intestine in the direction of most ease and holds it until there is a release. This same procedure is repeated in the RUQ, the LUQ, and the LLQ, in that order.

LIVER FLIP:

This procedure is performed to release a liver "entrapped" by the diaphragm; it frees the liver and aids in the decongestion of the right lung base and the superior portion of the liver. Too vigorous an application or a friable liver are contraindications to this procedure.

o .. The patient is supine; the operator stands on the right side of the patient.
o .. The operator's left hand is placed under the right rib cage about the level of the 6th, 7th and 8th ribs posteriorly and the right hand is placed on the anterior rib cage just superior to the anterior-inferior margin of the right rib cage at the mid-clavicular line.
o .. The patient is instructed to inhale deeply and follow this with a full exhalation; the operator's hand follows the rib cage down, compressing over the rib cage as the patient exhales.
o .. The compression is maintained as the patient is instructed to inhale deeply; as the rib cage elevates with forced inhalation, the operator suddenly releases the compression with the right hand. (The patient must have his/her mouth open during this procedure.)
o .. The procedure is repeated 2-3 times

BASIC LOCAL SOFT TISSUE TREATMENTS: kneading, stretching, massage and wringing of soft tissues.

EFFLEURAGE: moderately light stroking of skin and subcutaneous tissues to move lymph through their small vessels toward the heart. Treatment always employs a stroking from distal to proximal.

FASCIAL RELEASE TREATMENTS:

o .. Intrinsic Activation: determine direction of rotation of the tissues and then hold them in that direction until they release (indirect method); follow tissue balance as dictated by palpation.

o .. Direct Method Fascial Treatment: move tissues in the direction of restriction and hold the fascial plane at that barrier. Traction is usually used as the activator but if this is painful, compression is tried.

PETRISSAGE: (used to break fascial adhesions)

o .. grasp skin and subcutaneous tissues in the region of the adhesions; lift and twist them clockwise and then counter clockwise
o .. at the resistance barrier in each direction, have the patient take a deep breath and give a deep, explosive cough

(Continued with charts of ventral abdominal, fascial, and lymphatic treatments on page 227.)

IV. TREATMENT FOR PARASYMPATHETIC NERVOUS SYSTEM DYSFUNCTION:

The parasympathetics often seem to be overlooked in osteopathic manipulative management because the hypersympathetic and lymphatic dysfunctions seem to be more clinically evident and demanding. It also seems that there have been less research and clinical reports regarding the results of modifying systemic disease through manipulative influence upon the parasympathetic system.

Parasympathetic influence to the body viscera is supplied by cranial nerves III, VII, IX, and X, and by the parasympathetic outflow through the pelvic splanchnic nerves from S2, 3, and 4. Parasympathetic fibers synapse in the autonomic ganglia in the head (ciliary, sphenopalatine, otic, submandibular, submaxillary), the cervical ganglia of the uterus, and the myenteric (Auerbach's) and submucosal (Meissner's) plexuses of the GI tract.

The parasympathetic fibers from CN III supply the eye; CN IX and CN X supply the carotid body and carotid sinus. CN VII synapses in the sphenopalatine ganglion to supply the glands in the mucous membranes of the sinuses, pharynx, Eustachian tubes, and the lacrimal glands. CN X also supplies the GI tract distally to the transverse or right colon. The pelvic splanchnic nerves (S2,3,4) supply parasympathetic fibers to the left colon and pelvic organs. A more complete chart is found on pages 192 and 193.

A. TREATMENT THROUGH THE SPHENOPALATINE GANGLION:

The sphenopalatine ganglion is located in the sphenopalatine fossa of the skull. It hangs from the maxillary division of the trigeminal nerve and cannot be reached directly by the palpating finger. It may be reached indirectly, through the open mouth of the patient by influencing the fascias of the pterygopalatine muscles. These fascias then manipulate the sphenopalatine (the pterygopalatine) ganglion. Parasympathetic fibers reach this ganglion from the greater petrosal nerve, a branch from the geniculate ganglion of the VII cranial nerve.

o .. Purpose: Treatment encourages establishment of a more normal cellular ratio between the goblet and the ciliated columnar epithelial cells in the nasal and sinus epithelium. Parasympathetic impulses reduce the goblet cells and increase the proportion of ciliated columnar cells to thick mucus producing goblet cells. Parasympathetic activity is a primary influence in the production of a thin saliva-like nasal secretions.
o .. The operator passes a cotted finger over the molars of the upper jaw on one side, then lateral and posterior to the maxillary ridge.
o .. From there the finger is moved cephalad over the pterygoid plates (just posterior to the maxillary ridge) to the extent permitted by the buccal mucosa in the mouth.

o .. The patient is then asked to nod toward the palpating finger. Two or three
    repetitions on each side of the mouth will provide an adequate treatment
    by indirectly applying pressure on the ganglion through the fascias of the
    pterygoid muscles.
o .. Effective treatment is signaled by unilateral "tearing of the eye on the side
    of treatment" produced by effective stimulation of the lacrimal gland
    which shares the same parasympathetic nerve supply.

B. TREATMENT THROUGH VAGUS NERVE INFLUENCE:

o .. Purpose: to balance parasympathetic influence to viscera of the neck, heart,
    lungs, kidneys, and the glands and GI tract (excluding the left colon).
o .. Soft tissue, condylar decompression, and manipulation of specific somatic
    dysfunction of the occipitomastoid, OA, AA, and C2 joints will benefit
    parasympathetic influence through CN X.
o .. The vagus nerve may possibly be influenced by inhibitory pressure over the
    celiac and superior mesenteric collateral ganglia.

C. TREATMENT THROUGH PELVIC SPLANCHNIC INFLUENCE:

o .. Purpose: to balance parasympathetic influence to the viscera (left colon and
    pelvic areas).
o .. Direct inhibition to the inferior mesenteric ganglia influences
    parasympathetic supply to the left colon and pelvis.
o .. With the patient prone, the operator can place one hand over the sacrum
    and enforce its application with the other hand. Encouragement of the
    motion of the sacrum with respiration or the enhancement of the
    craniosacral motion will help to balance sacral splanchnic output.
    (Technique: Rocking the sacrum)
o .. With the patient supine, the operator can place one hand under the sacrum
    with the fingers directed cephalad and the sacral body resting in the palm
    of the operator. The operator senses the preference indicated by the
    craniosacral motion and follows this motion. Sometimes the operator's
    cephalad hand and forearm are placed across the two ASIS so they can
    be pulled toward approximation, to encourage separation of the
    sacroiliac joints and improve the realization and action of the
    craniosacral impulse.
o .. Treatment of sacral and innominate somatic dysfunction is also important.
    It is especially important to remove any non-physiologic sacral shear or
    superior innominate shear if present.

V. TREATMENT OF THE SOMATIC SYSTEM:

Spinal somatic dysfunction is especially important in the T1-L2 area. This is
true because dysfunction here can directly influence the cord segments

containing the primary sympathetic cell bodies by establishing facilitation of those divisions. It should be recognized that if there is a facilitated segment, somatic dysfunction anywhere may produce impulses that will cause that distant segment to fire. In general, the rotational component of the somatic dysfunction related to visceral dysfunction will usually be toward the same side as the organ, especially if that organ is paired. If there is a non-neutral segmental somatic dysfunction in an area it is more likely to influence or be connected with dysfunction of a organ connected to the sympathetic innervation at that cord level.

Treatment is designed to remove the somatic dysfunction and is based mainly upon the problem, the condition of the patient, and the skill of the physician. It must be stated that, clinically, high velocity, low amplitude methods of activation (HVLA) are often unsuccessful, especially when palpation of the paraspinal tissues has a "rubbery" texture.

VI. SUMMARY:

In most viscerosomatic reflexes, treatment of the visceral component with medications, diet, surgery, or some other modality is utilized if the structural component warrants that level of intervention. Treatment of the soma in a viscerosomatic reflex arc is often helpful in breaking this reflex cycle and is beneficial for the functional component. Reduction of stressors at physical, mental, spiritual, and environmental levels (etc.) is a great benefit as well, regardless of whether the primary problem is visceral or somatic.

In designing a manipulative approach in a patient with a facilitated segment, strongly consider removing this "neurologic lens" prior to instituting any other osteopathic manipulative treatment or introducing any other stressor. Recall that any osteopathic manipulative treatment will initially raise sympathetic tone slightly but will be followed by a clinically more important gradual, prolonged decline. The degree of rise will depend upon the amount of neurologic input. For this reason select the proper technique for the patient's condition. Remember that high velocity, low amplitude techniques will often be ineffective in removing somatic dysfunction that is secondary to visceral dysfunction and an alternative activating force must then be chosen.

––––––––––––

REFERENCES:

1. Patterson MM: Model mechanism for spinal segmental facilitation. <u>JAOA</u> Sept 1976; 76: 121-131.
    and Patterson MM: The reflex connection: History of a middleman. <u>Osteopathic Annals</u> Sept 1976; 357-367.
    and Patterson MM: Louisa Burns memorial lecture 1980: The spinal cord-- Active processor but not passive transmitter. <u>JAOA</u> Nov 1980; 80(3): 210-216.
2. Herrmann, Edward; <u>The D.O.</u> Oct 65; 163-164
3. Owens C <u>An Endocrine Interpretation of Chapman's Reflexes</u>. Carmel CA, 1963.
4. Kirksville College of Osteopathic Medicine; Department of Osteopathic Theory and Methods; 800 West Jefferson Street, Kirksville, Missouri 63501
5. Simons D.G., Travell JG: Myofascial origins of low back pain: Part 2. Torso muscles. <u>Postgraduate Medicine</u> February 1983; 73(2): 85-89.

TABLE: VENTRAL ABDOMINAL, FASCIAL RELEASE; LYMPHATIC PUMPS AND VISCERAL TREATMENTS

TECHNIQUE	PHYSIOLOGIC GOAL ATTEMPTED	INDICATIONS	CONTRAINDICATIONS
VENTRAL ABDOMINAL RX:			
Liver Flip (p 221)	free diaphragm; milk right lung base	decreased diaphragm motion; rales in right lower lobe	friable, enlarged liver
Celiac Ganglion Tension Release (pp 199-200)	calm sympathetics T5-9	upper GI dysfunction palpable subxiphoid tension	aortic aneurysm open surgical wound
Superior Mesenteric Ganglion Release (pp 199-200)	calm sympathetics T10-11	dysfunction of sm intestines below duodenum, right colon, upper GU; palpable tension midway between xiphoid and umbilicus	aortic aneurysm open surgical wound
Inferior Mesenteric Ganglion Release (pp 199-200)	calm sympathetics T12-L2	lower GI/pelvic dysfunction palpable tension just above the umbilicus	aortic aneurysm open surgical wound
Cecal Release (p 221)	improve bowel function (mechanical release)	complaints of constipation or RLQ pain of mechanical etiology; visceroptosis	appendiceal inflammation open surgical wound
Mesenteric Colon Release (Ascending/Descending) (p 221)	improve bowel function (mechanical release)	complaints of constipation of mechanical etiology	open surgical wound colitis
Mesenteric Small Intestinal Release (p 221)	improve bowel function (mechanical release)	abdominal cramping and/or tenderness; altered stool texture	open surgical wound

(continued)

TABLE: VENTRAL ABDOMINAL, FASCIAL RELEASE; LYMPHATIC PUMPS AND VISCERAL TREATMENTS   continued   B

TECHNIQUE	PHYSIOLOGIC GOAL ATTEMPTED	INDICATIONS	CONTRAINDICATIONS
VENTRAL ABDOMINAL cont.			
Abdominal Fascial Release (p 221)	to decrease intra-abdominal pressure; improve bowel function (mechanical)	abdominal tenderness; hernia	open surgical wound
Splenic Pump (p 219)	improve immune function	infection, fever	enlarged spleen, mononucleosis
Liver Pump (p 220)	detoxification; mobilize lymph	passive hepatomegaly, epigastric lymphatic congest. chronic toxic conditions	friable liver
(Ischiorectal Fossa) (pp 216-217)	improve pelvic diaphragm mobility; decongestion; reduce intra-abdominal press.	bloated feeling; hernia; lower extremity varicosities	perineal abscess (patient incontinence)
FASCIAL TREATMENTS:			
Rib Raising (pp 195-198)	improve lymphatic/venous return and immune function; calm sympathetic hyperactivity; improve thoracoabdominopelvic pump	visceral dysfunction; respiration not extending to pubic symphysis; tight paraspinal muscles; fever; lymphatic congestion	region of spinal fracture region of spinal surgery region of rib fracture(s) (pleurisy)
Redoming Thoracic Diaphragm (pp 215-216)	improve lymphatic/venous return and immune function	respiration not extending to pubic symphysis; lymphatic congestion (anywhere)	tubes, incisions, etc.

(continued)

TABLE: VENTRAL ABDOMINAL, FASCIAL RELEASE; LYMPHATIC PUMPS AND VISCERAL TREATMENTS (continued)

TECHNIQUE	PHYSIOLOGIC GOAL ATTEMPTED	INDICATIONS	CONTRAINDICATIONS
FASCIAL TREATMENTS cont.			
Intravaginal/Intrarectal Fascial Release (pp 216-217)	improve pelvic diaphragm motion; decongestion; decrease pelvic floor spasm	spasm of pelvic floor on vaginal and/or rectal exam; vaginitis, prostatic spasm; if poor results with ischiorectal fossa treatment	rectal or anal abscess rectal or anal malignancy
LYMPHATICS/LYMPH PUMPS:			
Liver Pump (see section "B" of this table) (p 220)	detoxification; mobilize lymphatic fluid	passive hepatomegaly; epigastric lymphatic congestion	friable liver
Lymphatic Pump (thoracic classic and rhythmic) (p 218)	accentuate negative intra-thoracic pressure; increase lymphatic return	rales and rhonchi; productive cough; lymphatic congestion; fever, infection	rib fracture; congestion too severe; incisions, subclavian lines etc. COPD unless Rx only at respiratory rate.
Lymphatic Pump: thoracic classic with vibratory modification (p 218)	same as above but uses vibratory component during pressure to loosen mucus	same; used in hopes of loosening plugs of mucus	same; (COPD patients only at intrinsic respiratory rate)
Lymphatic Pump: thoracic classic with accentu-ation of negative phase (p 218)	same as above; but during patient's inhalation, there is sudden release of thoracic pressure	same as above	loose dentures, gum, medication etc. in mouth
Pedal lymphatic Pump (pp 218-219)	accentuate negative intra-abdominal pressure; increase lymphatic return	may be able to use when thoracic pump can not; lymph congestion; fever; infection	venous thrombosis; lower extremity problems; abd. surgery (post-op)

229

(continued)

TABLE: VENTRAL ABDOMINAL, FASCIAL RELEASE; LYMPHATIC PUMPS AND VISCERAL TREATMENTS (continued)

TECHNIQUE	PHYSIOLOGIC GOAL ATTEMPTED	INDICATIONS	CONTRAINDICATIONS
LYMPHATIC/PUMPS cont.			
Lymphatic Pump (seated)	same as pedal pump	same as pedal pump congestion (anywhere)	unable to sit
Pectoral Traction (p 219)	accentuate negative intra-abdominal pressure; in-crease lymphatic/venous return	(can be taught to a family member); lymphatic congestion; fever; infection	tubes, lines, incisions on the chest
Posterior Axillary Fold (p 220)	increase lymph drainage from upper extremity; calm sympathetics T2-6; Rx for some myofascial points	shoulder dysfunction; hand and arm paresthesias; cool and clammy hand	excessive ticklishness
Breast "Drainage"	decrease lymphatic congestion of breast	Fibrocystic breasts; post-partum breast engorgement; breast tenderness	mastitis; malignancy in the breast
SPECIAL CLINICAL (OTHER)			
Fascial Release: cough activation (p 222)	break superficial and deep fascial adhesions	scar tissue adhesions; restricted range of motion	surgical wound or incision not completely healed
Ileus Prevention treat-ment: thoracolumbar inhibition (p 198)	decrease sympathetic hyperactivity to GI and restore normal bowel funct.	ileus or reduced bowel sounds; prevent ileus from recent surgery or planned	local infection; incision; thoracolumbar fracture

(continued)

TABLE: VENTRAL ABDOMINAL, FASCIAL RELEASE; LYMPHATIC PUMPS AND VISCERAL TREATMENTS   (continued)

TECHNIQUE	PHYSIOLOGIC GOAL ATTEMPTED	INDICATIONS	CONTRAINDICATIONS
SPECIAL CLINICAL cont.			
Sacral Inhibition (p 224)	improve parasympathetic activity in left colon; decongest uterus; calm hyper-parasympathetic activity; calm visceral afferents from left colon; reduce pain from cervical dilation (in labor)	Dysmenorrhea; make patient more comfortable in second and third stage of labor; Diarrhea; (constipation)	local infection; local incisions
Sphenopalatine Ganglion Treatment (pp 223)	thin mucosal secretion via parasympathetic influence	thick nasal secretions; nasal-lacrimal syndrome	trigeminal neuralgia; patient unable to cooperate, i.e. may bite you
Supra-/Infra-Orbital Treatment (p 28)	decrease sensitivity of visceral afferent receptors from mucous membranes of the head area	sinus headache; sinusitis; tenderness over the innervation of the supra- or infra-orbital nerves	neuritis of the supra- and infra-orbital nerves
Myofascial Spray and Stretch of Right Pectoralis Major (p 57)	decrease input to SA node from somatovisceral aff. to decrease supraventricular tachyarrhythmias	Supraventricular tachy-arrhythmias not responsive to usual medications in a patient with this trigger pt.	if unable to rule out primary cardiac disease or if have not treated the cardiac disease
Chapman's Reflex treatment (pp 200-201, 232-233)	decrease sympathetic tone produced by afferent visceral bombardment from soma to associated visceral tissues	history of symptoms of organ dysfunction; palpable Chapman myofascial point; other physical confirmation	

CHAPMAN'S REFLEXES: anterior points

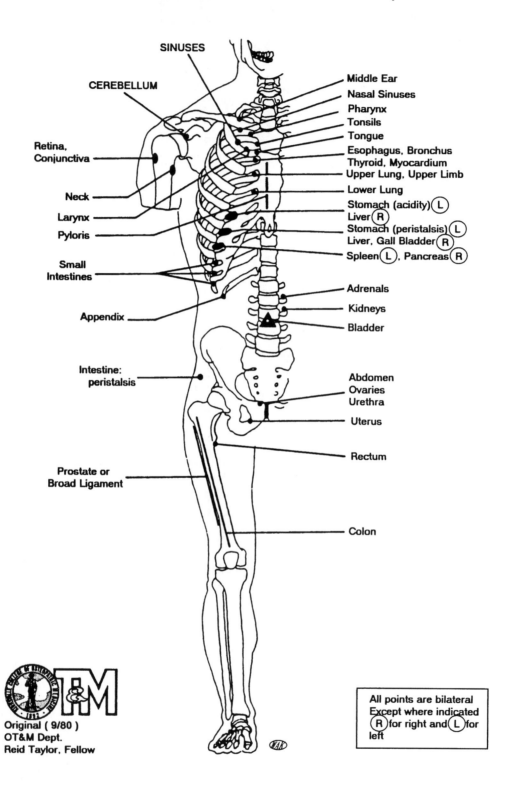

SINUSES

CEREBELLUM

Retina,
Conjunctiva

Neck

Larynx

Pyloris

Small
Intestines

Appendix

Intestine:
peristalsis

Prostate or
Broad Ligament

Middle Ear
Nasal Sinuses
Pharynx
Tonsils
Tongue
Esophagus, Bronchus
Thyroid, Myocardium
Upper Lung, Upper Limb
Lower Lung
Stomach (acidity) Ⓛ
Liver Ⓡ
Stomach (peristalsis) Ⓛ
Liver, Gall Bladder Ⓡ
Spleen Ⓛ, Pancreas Ⓡ

Adrenals
Kidneys
Bladder

Abdomen
Ovaries
Urethra
Uterus

Rectum

Colon

Original (9/80)
OT&M Dept.
Reid Taylor, Fellow

All points are bilateral
Except where indicated
Ⓡ for right and Ⓛ for
left

CHAPMAN'S REFLEXES: posterior points

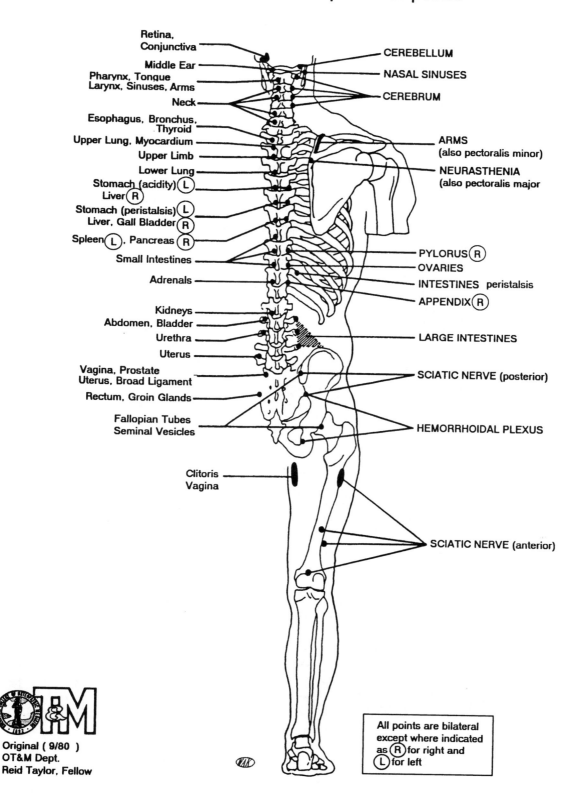

Retina, Conjunctiva
Middle Ear
Pharynx, Tongue
Larynx, Sinuses, Arms
Neck
Esophagus, Bronchus, Thyroid
Upper Lung, Myocardium
Upper Limb
Lower Lung
Stomach (acidity) (L)
Liver (R)
Stomach (peristalsis) (L)
Liver, Gall Bladder (R)
Spleen (L), Pancreas (R)
Small Intestines
Adrenals
Kidneys
Abdomen, Bladder
Urethra
Uterus
Vagina, Prostate
Uterus, Broad Ligament
Rectum, Groin Glands
Fallopian Tubes
Seminal Vesicles
Clitoris
Vagina

CEREBELLUM
NASAL SINUSES
CEREBRUM
ARMS (also pectoralis minor)
NEURASTHENIA (also pectoralis major
PYLORUS (R)
OVARIES
INTESTINES peristalsis
APPENDIX (R)
LARGE INTESTINES
SCIATIC NERVE (posterior)
HEMORRHOIDAL PLEXUS
SCIATIC NERVE (anterior)

All points are bilateral except where indicated as (R) for right and (L) for left

Original (9/80)
OT&M Dept.
Reid Taylor, Fellow

233

INDEX FOR OSTEOPATHIC MANIPULATIVE TECHNIQUES
IN SYSTEMIC DISEASE

CONTENTS

A

B

G

M

O

P

U